Surfing the Covid Waves

Anjan Kr Dasgupta
Prantar Chakrabarti

Powered by
24by7Publishing.com

This book **'Surfing the Covid Waves'** by Anjan Kr Dasgupta and Prantar Chakrabarti is self-published by the authors.

All the printing & distribution processes of the book
is powered by

24by7 Publishing
13 New Road, Kolkata - 51, India
https://www.24by7Publishing.com
mail@24by7publishing.com
+91 9831 470 133
+91 9433 444 334

Cover Design by Arko Dasgupta Srivastava

MRP: INR 249.00

First Published in February, 2025

Version 1.00

ISBN: 978-81-981020-1-0

Powered by

24by7Publishing.com

Foreward

COVID-19 infection is in many ways a turning point in our civilisation as many past epidemics had been. However Covid- 19 epidemic/pandemic is different from past events in many different ways. This pandemic happened in the full glare of electronic and other media which depicted the magnitude of human sufferings in all its dimensions. Economy of many countries were destroyed and the whole world economy went into near recession. Most advanced countries were found lacking in their ability to manage the thrust of the pandemic and modern medicine floundered. Drugs like hydroxychloroquine, ivermectin etc. took the place as a repurposed drug. Pharmaceutical industry worked overtime after going through their inventory of anti HIV drugs. Diagnosis of COVID infection also evolved using modern molecular biology tools. Epidemiologists got busy in understanding this pandemic.

Meanwhile the major question was how a bat virus jumped the species to produce it's pathogenicity to human beings. In natural conditions, such changes are known to be extremely rare raising the spectre of a possible human hand in creating such a monster. Theories were abound and several countries were suspected to have conspired to create such an organism as a biowar weapon which might have inadvertently or willingly leaked from the Wuhan Laboratory in China. To create such an organism mammoth funds and technological know how was needed.

While the whole world was under the grip of the pandemic,big pharmaceuticalhouses started competing with each other for producing vaccines against COVID using classical,cDNA,RNA technology. Many of these technologies were never proven on human beings, but looking at the global crisis, US FDA and other regulatory authorities gave permission to run abbreviated trials and market the vaccine. This allowed giant pharmaceuticals to test millions of human beings with hitherto unproven vaccine technology. Some of those vaccine have now been withdrawn for causing significant side effects, even death. However pharma companies learned their lessons on millions of humans with some of the future technologies.

Insurance companies also faced many challenges and some of them went bankrupt.

This book by Drs Chakrabarti and Dasgupta, has in an easily readable way painted the COVID-19 pandemic on a large canvas describing many of the dimensions of this infection affecting and threatening human society. I have found the book to be simply unputdownable and once one opens the first page then like a fast moving thriller one is glued upto its end asking for more.

The authors are experienced in Medicine and Biochemistry. In addition, Dr Chakrabarti with his experience on e-health technology has not only described the present crisis but has documented the lessons from it and outlined how humans may be able to avert a future crisis which possibly is not very far away.

I am very thankful to both the authors for giving me the opportunity to write a forward for this marvellous book. I wish this book all the success.

Prof Kanjaksha Ghosh. MBBS, MD,
MRCPI, FRCP(Glasg), FRCPath ((London), FAMS,
FACP(USA), FNASc, FICP, FFHom(London).

Former Director,

National Institute of Immunohaematology (ICMR).

Mumbai, India.

Table of Contents

List of Tables

List of Figures

The Story Behind the Scenes

Let us start with some personal notes from myself (ADG) and Dr. Prantar Chakrabarti (PC).

ADG: It was 2019 when my son went to Fudan University, Shanghai, China, to pursue Post Doctoral Research. All was well till he started complaining that he was getting the news of an unknown fever from his friends. Then came the winter holidays and suddenly he found all the shops closed. He rushed back to Kolkata.

> ⓘ Note
>
> It was a trying time for me as I had just retired from the Biochemistry Department of Calcutta University and was desperately looking for an engagement. The change of inertia from an extremely busy schedule to the idle lifestyle of a retired Professor created a great vacuum in me.

PC: When my late father suddenly resigned from his job (because of disagreements with the authority), my mother hardly knew that I would crack both the JEE entrance (Engineering and Medical). I had been fortunate enough to get an opportunity to play with a personal computer as early as 1987. I chose to pursue Medicine because I believed I would be more independent in my professional life. After MBBS, I got a taste of Kolkata's corporate sector before pursuing an MD in General Medicine. I had a brief stint in the Pollution Control Board and then was selected as a medical teacher. I decided to specialize in Clinical Hematology and obtained a DM from AIIMS, New Delhi.

> ⓘ Note
>
> Inside me, I always thought that I would do something different to touch people's lives. I worked in the government sector for 17 years and in the corporate sector for 3 years, and ultimately, I decided to resign from the post of Professor and Head of the Department of Hematology at NRS Medical College, Kolkata, in June 2019. I was looking for an alternative third model to build a team of dedicated healthcare providers who would provide quality and affordable care with significant empathy, outreach and community participation, incorporating digital health, data science and artificial intelligence using effective leadership and communication skills

The book is the outcome of a casual chat I had with ADG when I was returning from my private clinic.

A Coincidence

Both of us (ADG and PC) agreed that we should write a book. However, the burning question was what the topic should be. We thought of various topics. In fact, we also made some attempts to name the possible book. I remember a few of them. Smart Doctor, 101 things that you will never be taught in a medical school, How to be a good patient, Games Healthcare Industry play, The hidden algorithms in the medical practice and The Digital Health journey. While we spent months debating a suitable topic, COVID-19 came. We decided to jump into it and build a roadmap on how to tackle the next pandemic. We soon realized the topic was so vast and complex that we would burn our fingers in this book project. The matter was so heterogeneous and full of conflicting news that we almost stopped writing for months together. Three and a half years later, I was under the impression that the issue was dead and that there was no point in digging out the terrible memory here and everywhere else. Today I was listening to https://www.youtube .com/watch?v=W4cuCt8Idaw. It was a podcast by a Chinese lady named Lei. She elegantly summarized the COVID-19 timeline.

Timeline of COVID-19 Events (2019-2024)

Timeline of COVID-19 Events (2019-2024)

Year/Month	**Event Description**
2019	
November	Wuhan Institute of Virology
November 17	First case reported
December 26	Unexplained infection was first reported
Last week of December	SARS coronavirus identified
Last week of December	Chinese lady doctor arrested
2020	
January	Other doctors exposing the virulent nature of the virus were accused of spreading false information

Year/Month	Event Description
January 11	Center of Disease Control& Prevention (CDC) updated its Travel Health Notice (THN) system for person travelling to Wuhan
2021	
Throughout 2021	Power struggles in China; general belief that the epidemic was over
2022	
December 9	China attacks India in Ladakh while COVID infection was exploding
2023	
Throughout 2023	Analysis of the COVID story reveals a mix of mass social trauma, domestic politics, and geopolitics
2024	
Throughout 2024	Assassination attempts on President Trump followed by the news of his win over Biden, his chief contender

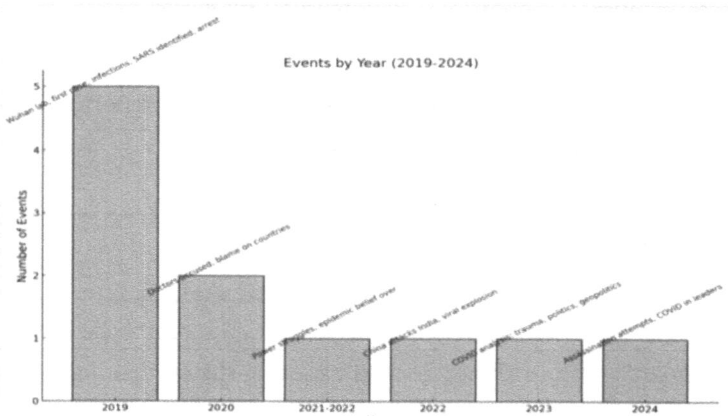

Events by year.

Now, it is 2024. We can see the big picture of how the COVID story evolved. On the one hand, it was a mass-scale social trauma that we have never witnessed before. On the other hand, the mix of domestic politics and geopolitics made the COVID stories intriguing. Every day, there was a report on the massive loss of life in some part of the world or the discovery of vaccines. Conspiracy theories like whether COVID is a geopolitical weapon also popped up. The news on the Wuhan lab leak from China or a gain of function research funding from the US occupied almost all news headlines. The supply chain disruption has caused a tsunami in geopolitics, with health departments restructuring in the US and worldwide.

- Was the outbreak due to an accidental leak from the Wuhan lab?
- How can we explain the role of WHO, which denied the possibility of person-to-person spread of the virus for a considerable time?
- How do you explain the roles of big pharma companies?
- Did they make a significant cross-section of human society as guinea pigs?
- After the re-explosion of the viral infection, where were we going?

It would be, thus, wise to explore COVID in view of the history of epidemics. The book highlights lessons to be learned from the COVID-19 pandemic that can help us prepare for future epidemics. While exploring different facets of the pandemic, we found that everything in the world is never purely good or bad. Even though the COVID-19 pandemic has been a terrible tragedy, it has also had some positive consequences. For example, it has led to an increase in our medical preparedness and readiness for eHealth and an increased interest in biomedical instrumentation. We may use a favourite quote often used by the co-author of this book, Prantar: "Fall in love with the problem and not the solution". The quote is attributed to Uri Levine, the co-founder of Waze and Moovit. The quote suggests that the best way to solve a problem is to understand the problem deeply and to be passionate about finding a solution. The book connects the dots between the COVID-19 pandemic, the history of epidemics, and the importance of understanding the problem before finding a solution. Incidentally, the phrase has been used by other entrepreneurs like Steve Blank: "The best entrepreneurs are obsessed with the problem, not the solution." Josh Linkner: "If you are solving a problem that no one cares about, you are going to have a hard time succeeding," Peter Thiel: "The best way to predict the future is to create it".

> ⓘ Note
>
> Fall in love with the problem and not the solution
> - Uri Levine

Lastly, we would like to quote from <https://www.cdc.gov/coronavirus/2019-ncov/covid-data /covidview/index.html>. The PHE public health emergency on May 2023 declared the end of the COVID-19 emergency. We started the book when COVID-19 just started. We hoped to complete the book when the emergency was over. We are in the winter of 2024, but there are reports of fresh COVID-19 outbreaks in China and other parts of the world. Astra Zeneca has acknowledged the fact that they were aware of VITT (Vaccine-induced Immune Thrombotic Thrombocytopenia), and legal proceedings continue (1). If we wait for the complete elimination of this deadly viral disease, we may never complete the book. Hence, we are gearing ourselves up to go ahead with the book as the loop of the pandemic outbreak, and its deceptive disappearance may continue for some time to come. We have also attempted to frame out the chaos that followed the pandemic in domestic events and geopolitics and have also tried to highlight the order that came out of the chaos.

An order out of chaos

It is easy to comprehend the disruption caused by COVID-19 in almost all spheres of life. However, we call it an "order out of chaos" because it taught us resilience, the ability to survive and grow under extreme disruptions. For instance, old Doordarshan episodes like Ramayana and Mahabharata broke viewership records with repeat broadcasts, offering comfort and nostalgia during the lockdown. There was also a significant boom in online courses across various educational institutions, marking a shift in learning paradigms.

The "work from home" culture became the norm rather than the exception, while many infrastructural projects benefited from reduced traffic. Railways and roadways were temporarily closed, allowing for maintenance and testing of new technologies to enhance future performance. Additionally, several governments, including India, legalized online medical consultations, enabling accessible healthcare from home. Policymakers also introduced innovative measures to mitigate supply chain disruptions, ensuring that essential goods reach the public effectively.

Acknowledgements

As we did not publicize writing this book, it was impossible for us to get suggestions from anyone on how to improve it. However, we must thank Dr Barnali Bhattacharyya for preparing the book's essential illustrations and plots. We also thank Panini (son of ADG, Postdoctoral Researcher, Seoul National University, Republic of Korea) for helping us with proofreading. We thank Dr Archit Pandharipande, Pediatric & Adult Hematologist-oncologist, BMT Physician for his valuable suggestions. We thank Arko Dasgupta Srivastava (BFA film making) for covert art and illustration.

1.
Why this Book?

The book deals with a bird's eye view of the corona-inflicted world. Our worldview, family relations, well-being, love of nature, love for neighbors, politics, social relationships, everything has been directly or indirectly affected by this pandemic. Interestingly, while our discussions regarding the book plan started at the beginning of 2019, the global disaster, particularly the so-called third wave, its attenuation in most parts of the world, its reemergence in some places (e.g., China), the significant social media upsurge on the effects of the vaccine, changed the world so much that we were at a loss on what to focus on the book. Briefly, in the initial period, we were almost running a commentary on a hotly contested match, a game between life and death. At the present stage, COVID-19 has stabilized, and some countries like Japan are considering downgrading the COVID-19 emergency to the level of flu. However, this unforgettable period should be narrated from multiple perspectives. As COVID has enriched the contents of scientific journals with a long list of literature, we wanted to highlight what a typical journal author never dares to mention. The socio-political impact was so enormous that this is undoubtedly going to invade the media and literature of the future in a more significant way than we can expect at present.

For example, India has a large and growing population, which makes it difficult to contain the spread of the virus. India also has a large informal economy, meaning many workers are not covered by social security or other forms of protection, which makes it difficult for people to cope with the economic losses caused by the pandemic.

The facts also point out that predicting the exact trajectory of a pandemic is challenging because pandemics are complex phenomena that are influenced by a variety of factors, including the behavior of human populations, the mutation of viruses, and the effectiveness of public health measures.

> ⓘ Note
>
> Let us now inspect data from WHO from April 2020 to May 2024

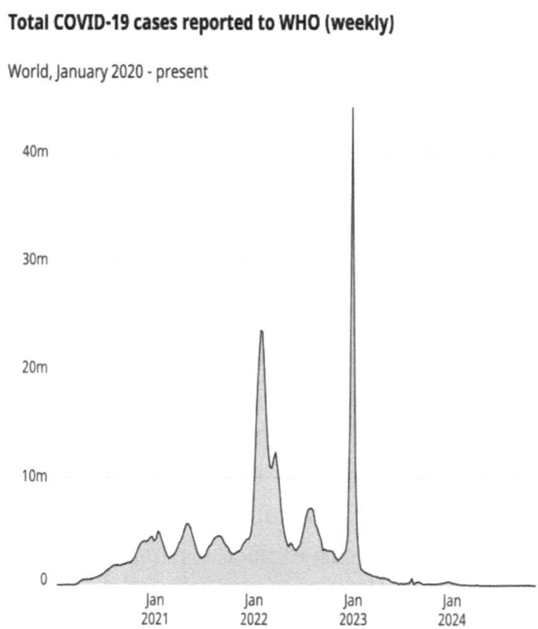

Figure 1.1 Year wise COVID death from 2019-2024

1.1 The Indian lesson from crisis

Crisis, as some people say, is the mother of invention. One sphere that realigned and developed from this crisis is eHealth. In India, especially post-COVID-19 pandemic, digital transformation of healthcare is currently the hottest topic and the highest priority for all involved stakeholders: governments, ministries and public authorities, healthcare providers, physicians and nurses, and, of course, patients and consumers. Consequently, Digital health domain specialists will be among the most demanded professionals in the coming years and decades. In conclusion, eHealth has been an essential tool in the fight against COVID-19, enabling healthcare providers to deliver care to patients safely and efficiently and providing the public with access to critical information and resources during the pandemic. A vaccine digital certificate, also known as an "e-vaccination certificate" or "vaccine passport," is an electronic document verifying that an individual has received a vaccine. In India, the government had launched an initiative to provide digital certificates for citizens who had received COVID-19 vaccines.

> ⓘ Note
>
> The digital certificate is stored in a government-backed platform, can be accessed by individuals through the Cowin app or a government website. It contains information such as the individual's name, date of birth, vaccine type, and date of vaccination.

The vaccine digital certificate aims to provide a secure and convenient way for individuals to prove their vaccination status, which can be helpful in various settings such as international travel, returning to work, or attending public events. It is also expected to help with the management of the vaccine rollout by enabling health authorities to track who has been vaccinated and monitor vaccine coverage rates. It is important to note that while the vaccine digital certificate is being encouraged to promote vaccination and help control the spread of COVID-19, it is not mandatory, and individuals have the right to choose whether to receive a vaccine and obtain a digital certificate.

1.2 First impression from a crowded metro in India

After the lockdown announcement, Kolkata Metro has not seen a prolonged closure since its beginning. Similarly, we have hardly witnessed barber shops, football grounds, religious places, or international airways closed for so many days. A young teenager confined to a room, taking online classes, and not in touch with friends is a situation occurring for the first time, the impact of which will only be realized in the future. Among the acute emergencies in all spheres of life, we found that the political discourses continued in democracies like India. While the COVID-19 crisis was being tackled, the Ukraine war broke out, plunging the world into another crisis, such as energy shortage.

1.3 COVID-specific eHealth challenges in the insurance sector

eHealth refers to using digital technologies to support and improve health and healthcare. During the COVID-19 pandemic, eHealth has played a crucial role in addressing some of the challenges posed by the virus. One of the critical ways eHealth has been utilized is through telemedicine, which allows patients to have virtual consultations with healthcare providers without having to physically visit a clinic or hospital. This has helped to reduce the spread of COVID-19 by reducing the number of people who need to be physically present in healthcare settings. It has also made it easier for people to access medical care from the safety of their homes. Another way eHealth has been used during the pandemic is by creating digital tools for tracking the spread of COVID-19, which has included the development of contact tracing apps, as well as websites and portals for monitoring the latest COVID-19 cases, deaths, and recovery rates. eHealth has also played a role in the distribution of vaccines against COVID-19. Many countries have set up digital platforms for booking vaccine appointments, as well as for tracking the progress of vaccine campaigns and monitoring vaccine safety.

Let us have a look at the impact of the pandemic on the insurance sector.

> ⓘ Note
>
> - Minimized physical visits to a clinic or hospital, which also reduced the spread of COVID-19
> - Invention of digital tools for tracking contact tracing apps
> - eHealth has also played a role in the distribution of vaccines against COVID-19

- **Increased demand for health insurance**: The pandemic has highlighted the importance of health insurance, leading to increased demand for health insurance products. Many individuals who did not previously have health insurance have taken out policies to protect themselves and their families in the event of a COVID-19 infection.
- **Changes in underwriting criteria**: To manage the risk posed by the pandemic, insurance companies have revised their underwriting criteria for health insurance. For example, certain insurance companies may now refuse to offer coverage to individuals with pre-existing conditions or may charge higher premiums for such individuals.
- **Impact on life insurance**: The pandemic has also impacted the life insurance sector. With many people losing their jobs and facing financial uncertainty, the demand for life insurance products has decreased. At the same time, the number of claims related to COVID-19 has increased, putting pressure on insurance companies to pay out large sums quickly.

- **Changes in claims management**: Insurance companies have had to adapt to the changing landscape by implementing new procedures for managing claims related to COVID-19. This has included the use of telemedicine and remote evaluation to assess claims, as well as the use of digital platforms for processing claims.
- **Impact on reinsurance**: The insurance industry is heavily reliant on reinsurance, which provides a safety net for insurance companies in the event of a large number of claims. The COVID-19 pandemic has put pressure on reinsurance companies, which have had to pay out large sums in a short period.

Overall, the COVID-19 pandemic has disrupted the insurance sector and has led to significant changes in the way insurance companies operate. While the industry has adapted to these challenges, the full impact of the pandemic is unlikely to be fully understood for some time.

1.4 Questions that popped out during our casual book-plan

It was a sheer coincidence that when we first planned this book, we never knew that the pandemic would make the eHealth issue so much more contextual. Among many popular theories, a post on Facebook became viral, namely pandemics like COVID-19 strike with eerie precision, every 100 years. For example, in 1720, there was the Plague; in 1820, a Cholera outbreak; in 1920, the Spanish Flu; and in 2020, the outbreak of the coronavirus. However, the fact check showed that the stated periodicity was false. The Plague cited was not a pandemic. According to the Statesman network fact check (which is slightly better than Deshi fact checks work in India, https:// www.statesman.com/ news/20200410/fact-check-has-pandemic-occurred-every-100-years), the pandemics did not occur exactly in the cited years; and, most importantly, numerous other pandemics have occurred without such synchronicity.

"I am suspicious of the idea that pandemics operate to a railroad timetable," Yale University history professor Frank Snowden, author of "Epidemics and Society," told PolitiFact, noting several problems with the post.

With all these fancy and often fake posts hanging around, we focused our discussions on specific relations between eHealth management and pandemics. The medical care systems in the world's most advanced countries appeared primitive.

The other reason this pandemic is unlike any previous instances of large-scale disease outbreaks (except for SARS or AIDS) is that the world has never been so small or this mobile.

1.5 Data data everywhere and nowhere

"Water, water, everywhere,

Nor any drop to drink."

The Rime of the Ancient Mariner

–Samuel Coleridge.

eHealth, which may have several synonyms, essentially is a balanced super-set of Data Science and Information, Communications and Technology(ICT). These two, backed up by suitable models, are the oft-used "invisible hands" that set the trends. Healthcare organizations use AI to automate processes, screen and e-inform patients using suitable messaging devices, and help manage supply chains. In the future, human-machine collaboration will permeate every aspect of every organization, enabling the reinvention of healthcare delivery.

In the health and drug research domain, AI applications, for example, are considered as potential but as dangerous as "self-driving cars".

Unlike bioinformatics, which is based on ordered and annotated data and has mainly indirect predictive abilities, eHealth has direct implications in wet clinical laboratories. Unlike bioinformatics, a small prediction error may cause loss of human life, which is more fatal than a crash of a "self-driving car". An example that is often cited is as follows. A programming error in a smart pacemaker by a reputed manufacturer caused numerous losses in life, and FDA approval was withdrawn for that model.

1.6 Data versus the model - Content and Form

The tremendous challenge a data scientist faces is often not an absence of data. Following Coleridge, we may say "data, data everywhere", but not a drop left for "analytics". Data is the new "gold/oil" reserve of the advanced world

Several laboratories from the West took the initiative to keep digital data records, perhaps anticipating the emergence of some future data-based commodities. Many pharma companies indeed used data as a commodity, and data on health and clinical records became subjects of hot extreme political and rights-issue-based debate.

In contrast, we have a poor record of book-keeping data. Unless health data is aggregated and organized, the dream of eHealth will be far-fetched. Even professional journals were not exceptions, with misleading reporting on hydroxychloroquine being a good example.

The model and data are often as closely related as a molecule's structure and function or any language's form and content. Quoting Kalidasa: "वागर्थविव समारितम वागर्थः प्रतिपत्तये" (Vagarthaviva samaritan vagarthah pratipattaye) where he highlighted the inseparability of speech and its meaning, we have similar entanglement between data and model. The effort raises some insights into this interplay, particularly in the context of health issues and managing a pandemic-like scenario.

1.7 Pandemic versus the infodemic

The COVID-19 pandemic was followed by an "*infodemic*", particularly on social media platforms. Out of many posts that became viral, one sounded highly convincing. This is because there is a re-occurrence of similar pandemics every 100 years. With an abundance of flashy and often misleading posts circulating online, the effect on the general public was, to say the least, "synergistic." On the one hand, people grappled with the suffering caused by the virus itself; on the other, they were bombarded with theories about the pandemic's history and origin, relentlessly propagated through popular social media platforms. While it is common for Western media to highlight COVID-19 mismanagement in third-world countries, the stark reality was that healthcare systems in even the most advanced nations often appeared alarmingly inadequate. The blame game among political parties—and even between nations—further exacerbated the situation.

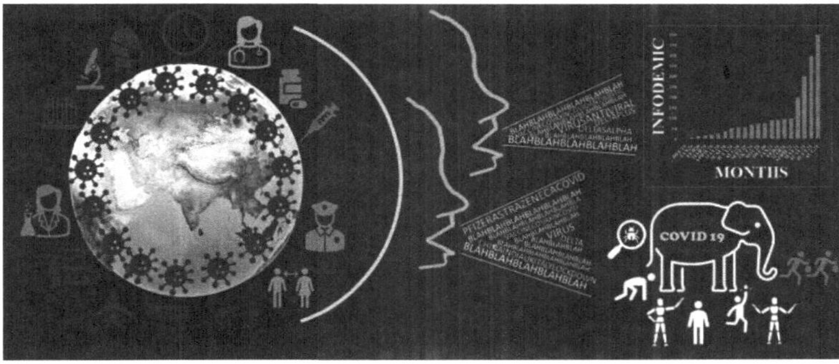

Figure 1.2 Cartoon illustrating the limitations in understanding the pandemic

1.8 Epidemics in fiction and movies

Plagues and pandemics have always added to the imagination of fiction writers. One of the earliest books on this theme is "A Journal of the Plague Year" (2). The author Defoe was only five when the Great Plague struck the city of London in the year 1665. There is, however, some debate on whether the book is an actual historical account of the bubonic Plague or if it was a fruit of imagination. The book Pox Americana (3) accounts for the disease that transformed the United States at its birth. Interestingly, this was the time when the American Revolution took place. Another book (4) describes the collapse of the long history of the Native American people by imported diseases. Another eminent book on pandemics is "The Plague" by Albert Camus" (5). The book describes townspeople in the grid of a deadly plague. Interestingly, Camus's novel is about individual determination against the precariousness of human existence.

Contemporary COVID-19 also competes with such historical literature on pandemics. Starting in 2020, there has been a burst of publications on pandemic books. Some notable fiction books on pandemics are "Breathtaking: Inside the NHS in a Time of Pandemic" (6). Several other books, "Vaxxers: The Inside Story of the Oxford AstraZeneca Vaccine and the Race Against the Virus" (7). The authors describe the inside story of the AstraZeneca book as a race, not against other vaccines but the deadly virus COVID-19. There are books with different flavours, e.g. (8) Our book deals with a bird's eye view of the new corona-inflicted world. We have attempted to touch upon the worldview, family relations, love for neighbours, social relationships, health workers' fate, and everything directly or indirectly affected by this pandemic. Interestingly, while our discussions regarding the book plan started, the so-called second or third wave (9,10) was a matter of great concern. Our self-confidence in dealing with medical emergencies, financial and other infrastructure matters, our social security concerns, and the livelihood of the vulnerable section of our society have suddenly come to a gigantic challenge not witnessed earlier. Perhaps we need to rethink and plan everything, including our approach to education, differently. The book deals with a scaffold of some such concerns.

There indeed may have been more, and the extinction of many unknown civilizations or animal species is excluded as we have yet to have direct proof in our hands. The extinction of the main Harappan civilization from its original location might have been caused by epidemics; however, this hypothesis remains purely conjectural, as there are numerous controversies surrounding the civilization's decline. Similarly, many researchers account for the extinction of Neanderthals or Denisovans (who were human-like and ruled the world for a very long time) by a sudden occurrence of epidemics in the past. The site https://www.visualcapitalist.com/history-of-pandemics-deadliest/ provides a detail of the reported pandemics with some more details.

How the consequences of Pandemics were actually translated into literature and movies? How the realization of such time bomb-like events has shaped our fiction and even our cultural ethos may be worth mentioning in this context. The 50-year-old film "The Andromeda Strain", which described a pandemic caused by a pathogen of extraterrestrial origin, or the Nobel prize-winning book (11) may be interesting examples of such cross-discipline realization of a pandemic-like situation. The novel The End of Men (12) is about a virus to which women are immune and kills 90% of the world's men. The author, Christina Sweeney-Baird, was shocked when she saw the resemblance between what she wrote in that book in 2018-2019 and what was happening during the COVID-19 pandemic just after that. The countries in that novel closed their borders, and doctors were helpless because their advice was not taken. Her objective was to show what the world of 'Men without women, the brainchild of Hemingway (13), would look like. Again, Steven Soderbergh's 2011 film Contagion (14) became one of the most-watched movies on the internet. While the film's fictional virus MEV-1, had a 72-hour incubation period and a much higher fatality rate than the present predictions regarding the coronavirus, the similarity of the scenes of this decade-old movie with the present scenario made it a top hit, the 10th-most-rented movie on iTunes. Other movies like

Station Eleven (15) describe how a virus kills an entire population and how it breaks down as a consequence of that. Severance by Ling Ma (16) tells the haunting story of "Shen fever", a fungus that originates in Shenzen and leaves sufferers technically alive but unaware of their existence. The speciality of this book (and movie) is the China connection and a particular reference to how the state media in China controls the optics of this. The Eyes of Darkness (17), Lastly we will end this section with a question. Why do such fiction writers imagine such situations at all? We are what our dreams are. We have been able to fly and go to space because of such dreams. We expected some fiction or movies on vaccine hesitancy and the sociopolitical origin of such trends. On the contrary, A new documentary, Medical Racism: The New Apartheid (a 57-minute film), has appeared, which is an advocacy piece for anti-vaxxers.

Table 1.1 Movies on pandemics.

Movie	Year	Director
Contagion	2011	Steven Soderbergh
Severance	2018	Ben Wheatley
Station Eleven	2020	Hiro Murai
The Eyes of Darkness	2021	Kimble Rendall
The End of Men	2021	Chloe Okuno
The Vaccine War	2023	Vivek Agnihotri

Table 1.2 Books on pandemics

Book	**Author**	**Year**
A Journal of the Plague Year	Daniel Defoe	1722
The Plague	Albert Camus	1947
Blindness	José Saramago	1995
Pox Americana	Stephen R. Fenn	2002
Severance	Ling Ma	2018
The End of Men	Christina Sweeney-Baird	2021
Breathtaking: Inside the NHS in a Time of Pandemic	Amanda Jane Robinson	2021
Vaxxers: The Inside Story of the Oxford AstraZeneca Vaccine and the Race Against the Virus	Sarah Gilbert and Catherine Green	2021

Meanwhile, we can look at the table, which provides the timelines of some historically recorded pandemics.

1.9 A brief account of the history of epidemics

Table 1.3 A brief history of epidemics

AD	Pandemic Description
541-542	Plague of Justinian
1346-1350	The Black
1899-1923	Cholera
1918-1923	Spanish Flu
1957-1958	Asian Flu (H2N2)
1968-1969	Hong Kong Flu
2009-2010	Swine Flu
2020-2021	COVID-19

There is, interestingly, no text on large-scale epidemics in the Indian subcontinent in ancient times. According to "The Encyclopedia Britannica", long back, it was a maxim that the Plague never appeared east of the Indus River. The third great plague pandemic in the world that spread from China in the late 19th century came to India on a ship to Bombay in 1896, and from there, it spread to the rest of India. India accounted for 95% of the worldwide fatalities. The other epidemics that followed occurred in India in the post-colonial time. The article (18) explains why smallpox, known as Masurika in Charak (and spring disease in eastern India), although known, never took an epidemic scale. Some traditional measures akin to vaccination were known, and the author cites the correspondence of the British lady Mary (19) to her friend Sarah Chiswell, who was infected by smallpox, regarding the indigenous prevention technique. A similar correspondence between Dr. Robercoult and another Englishman regarding the local treatment of smallpox is also noted. The local practice bore striking similarities to the fundamental concept of modern vaccine production. The other report that has appeared in the recent epidemic literature is the possibility of mass extinction of the Harappan population after the onset of an epidemic (20). The authors mention that although climate changes and high levels of urbanization might have caused diseases like tuberculosis or leprosy, they did not have the answer to whether there was a mass extinction of the Harappan population. The question that often circulates in private circles of historians is whether an epidemic-like situation caused the sudden disappearance of this highly urbanized civilization. The contrasting claim that may be raised is that there were no mass graves or funeral sites. The other contrasting evidence that the Harappan population got mixed with the other population from the rest of India stems from the striking similarity of the Harappan artefacts with folk crafts or sculptures obtained from remote villages in Rajasthan and other places. The absence of evidence (e.g. the linguistic scripture) elsewhere makes this debate even more intense. However, the Harappan extinction process summarizes that it is unlikely that an epidemic caused such a catastrophic event. We are yet to realize whether it was a catastrophic episode or a gradual process where a population with a high degree of urbanization gets mixed up with its neighboring population.

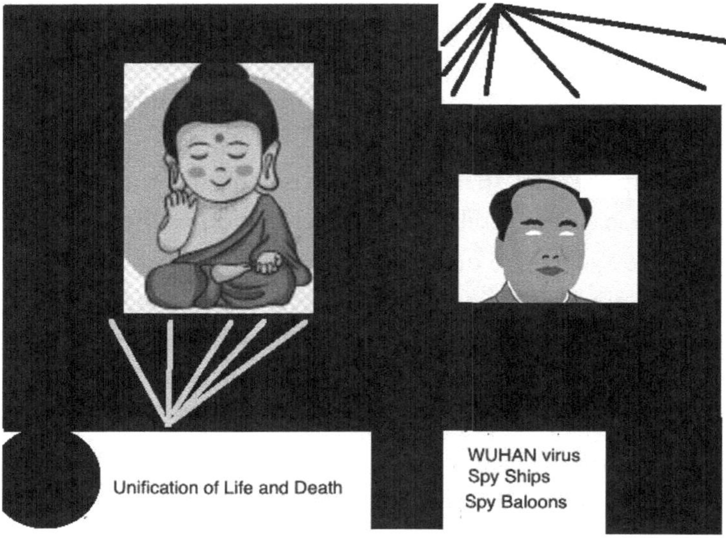

Figure 1.3 Two narratives

1.10 The Cycle of Information and Disinformation

It was a full circle moment as Dr David Martin informed 16 members of the UK Parliament that COVID was a 56-year plan in the making, which started in the UK when the Welcome Trust decided to use the corona as the "preferred form of human manipulation". The so-called Gates Plan. The UK's most decorated oncologist/immunologist tells cancer specialists at the RAD51 conference that the COVID mRNA vaccine safe and effective mantra is "a BIG LIE". Prof Angus Dalgleish presents data exposing that boosters are accelerating cancer.

Elon Musk wrote on X, "Have you heard of this disinformation?" He wrote this in a play on words, captioning a video he shared on September 26, 2023. As per details, the clip was a montage of 111 screenshots of headlines, scientific article titles, and websites that purport to show diminishing levels of protection over time from vaccines against COVID-19. Apart from this, this also highlights percentages in red in the text on the screen, giving the impression as the video progresses that confidence in the effectiveness of the vaccine has degraded throughout the rollout of the shots, said the report. Details say Musk did not create the video, but it was already circulated on social media already in November 2022.

However, interest in the clip following the post of the tech billionaire who bought Twitter in 2022 generated more than 635,800 likes and 197,300 reposts as of October 18.

Emily Kopp a US reporter who investigated the pandemic tweeted "*EcoHealth Alliance's response to my story does not actually include any "false statements," which is why they dodged my questions and didn't say anything until after the story published. The statement argues that DEFUSE wasn't funded so it shouldn't matter that EcoHealth lied to DARPA and has been lying to the public for years. I disagree.*"

2.
Epidemiology as a Scientific Discipline

Epidemiology is a scientific discipline involved in studying the spread and causal factors of 'health-related states or events' in different populations and the exertion of the study for control of health problems. Needless to say, epidemiology forms the backbone of public health.

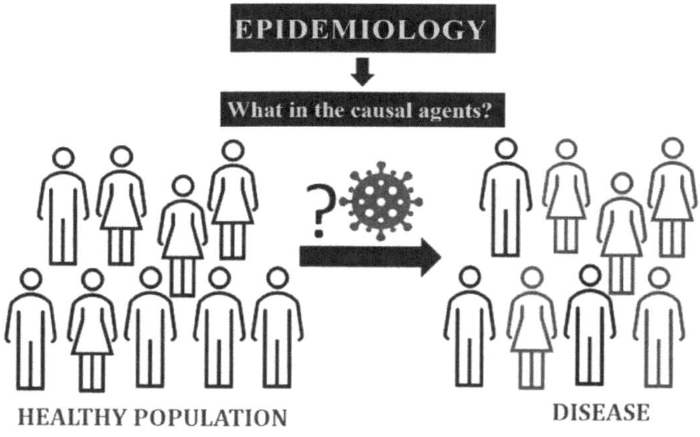

Figure 2.1 Epidemiology

Epidemiology is the study of the distribution and determinants of disease in populations. It is a scientific discipline that uses methods from statistics, biology, and other fields to investigate the patterns, causes, and effects of health and disease. Epidemiologists use their findings to help prevent and control disease, improve health, and make policy decisions.

Epidemiology is a broad field with many different areas of specialization within it. Some of the most common areas of specialization include:

- **Infectious disease epidemiology**: This area of epidemiology focuses on studying infectious diseases. Epidemiologists in this area study how infectious diseases spread, how to prevent them, and how to treat them.
- **Cancer epidemiology**: This area focuses on the study of cancer. Epidemiologists in this area study the causes of cancer, how to prevent it, and how to treat it.
- **Environmental epidemiology**: This area focuses on studying the relationship between environmental factors and health. Epidemiologists in this area study how environmental factors, such as air pollution, water pollution, and chemical exposure, can affect health.
- **Occupational epidemiology**: This area of epidemiology focuses on studying the relationship between work and health. Epidemiologists in this area study how workplace hazards, such as exposure to chemicals or noise, can affect health.

2.1 Formal Definitions

The general population seems to be reading, listening and talking about terms like pandemic, infectious disease, virus, antibody tests, SARS-CoV-2, variants of concern and vaccine efficacy fervently like religious scriptures. However, in a 'warlike' situation like this, it is best to begin with the very beginning by brushing up a few definitions before we delve into a disease that has stolen the limelight as a 'pandemic'.

As per the dictionary, the term "demic" represents people or population. Parasites, fungi, bacteria and viruses preceded humans in the evolutionary tree. There has been crosstalk between these species throughout human existence. Many believe that the extinction of certain predecessors of human-like mammals like the Neanderthals (21) was caused by a loss of species equilibrium (between bacteria, viruses and the host cells). In other words, they were extinct, as the infectious interactions defeated the normal cellular metabolism. To exemplify, we may cite an important lesson from the history of disease. Bubonic plague and smallpox caused the Hittle and Carthaginian empires to end. In fact, the book (22) argues that infectious disease epidemics are critical links to the chain of events that caused the demise of many civilizations in the ancient world.

There are other books covering different socio-political scenarios during the pandemic. For example, the pandemic association of Cuban independence is described in (23). How the world of the 1918 influenza epidemic is described in (24). How the ignored tropical disease affects the continents of Africa and Asia is depicted in (25). The book (26) focuses on the 'Disease, politics of starvation and the loss of Aboriginal life'. One of the books on the 'Faith, Reason, and the Plague' may also be cited here (27). A book recently published on the overall history of pandemics is (28).

Let us now define the terms Endemic, Epidemic and Pandemic. Endemic refers to a disease localized in a certain class of population, which may include chicken pox, which occurs at a predictable rate among young school children in the United States and India, and malaria in some areas of Africa and the Indian subcontinent. An epidemic is an outbreak that affects a large population at a given time. One of the classic examples is the cholera epidemic. A pandemic is a class of epidemic whose spread is global. The virus that is likely to have Wuhan origin (COVID-19) was initially thought to be associated with epidemics in specific locations in the globe. It is only since March 2020 that the WHO has termed COVID-19 a pandemic due to its global spread.

However, while a clinician focuses on treating a disease in an individual or small group of individuals, an epidemiologist's concern is the health of an entire epidemiological triad (Figure 2.2). A simple model of infectious disease causation is represented by a triad comprising three components: the agent (in this case, SARS-CoV-2), the susceptible host (bats, pangolins, or humans), and the environment where these elements interact (https://www.cdc.gov/). This concept aligns with the simplest model for epidemics, the SIR model (Susceptible-Infectious-Recovered), as described by Duggan and Northeastern Illinois University. University Honors Program (1998).

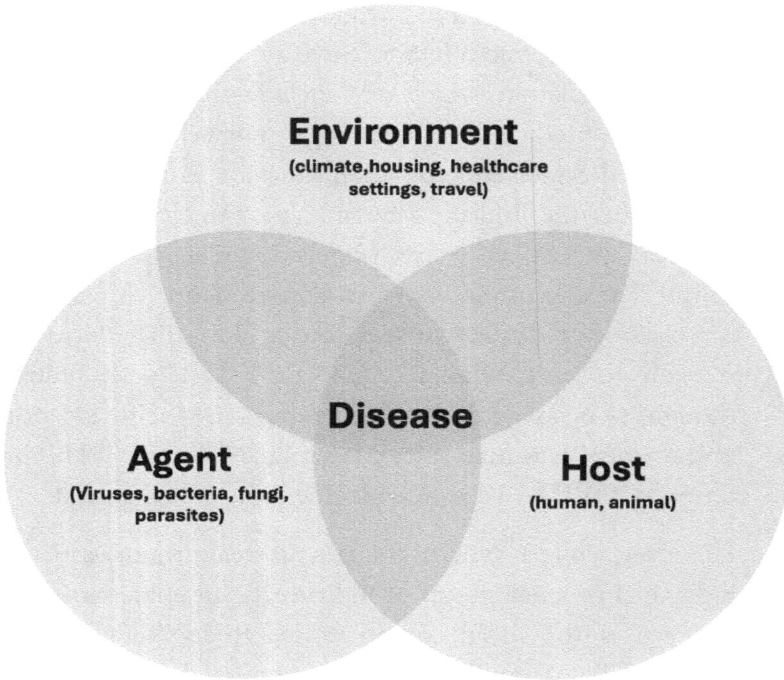

Figure 2.2 Epidemiological Triad

Table 2.1 Classes of epidemics

Term	Definition	Example
Endemic	A disease that is localized in a certain class of population.	Chicken pox occurs at a predictable rate among young school children in the United States and India, and malaria in some areas of Africa and the Indian subcontinent.
Epidemic	An outbreak that affects a large population at a given time.	The cholera epidemic.
Pandemic	That class of epidemic whose spread is global.	COVID-19.
Agent	The pathogen that causes the disease.	SARS-CoV-2.
Host	The organism that is infected with the pathogen.	Humans, bats, pangolins.
Environment	The physical and social conditions in which the pathogen and host interact.	The place where the pathogen and host come together, such as a hospital, a school, or a community.

2.2 SIR model - the simple harmonic oscillator of epidemics

The reference (29) provides some details of the SIR model, a basic conceptual framework to understand epidemics. The model is expressible by the following sets of ODES (ordinary differential equations).

$$\frac{dS}{dt} = -\beta S \cdot I/N \tag{2.1}$$

$$\frac{dI}{dt} = -\beta S \cdot I/N \tag{2.2}$$

$$\frac{dR}{dt} = \gamma I. \tag{2.3}$$

where, $N = S + I + R$

SIR model (Duggan and Northeastern Illinois University. University Honors Program, 1998). While the R number is popular among news media and common biological researchers and epidemiologists, the simplest model is slightly more involved as it involves three groups (susceptible S, infected I and recovered R). The SIR model can be expressed by the differential equations expressed in the following code:

```
library(deSolve)
library(tidyverse)

closed.sir.model <- function (t, x, params) {
  ## first extract the state variables
  S <- x[1]
  I <- x[2]
  R <- x[3]
```

```
  ## now extract the parameters
  beta <- params["beta"]
  gamma <- params["gamma"]
  N <- S+I+R
  ## now code the model equations
  dSdt <- -beta*S*I/N
  dIdt <- beta*S*I/N-gamma*I
  dRdt <- gamma*I
  ## combine results into a single vector
  dxdt <- c(dSdt,dIdt,dRdt)
  ## return result as a list!
  list(dxdt)
}

parms <- c(beta=400,gamma=365/13)

times <- seq(from=0,to=60/365,by=1/365/4)
xstart <- c(S=999,I=1,R=0)
ode(
  func=closed.sir.model,
  y=xstart,
  times=times,
  parms=parms
) %>%
  as.data.frame() -> out
out %>%
gather(variable,value,-time) %>%
ggplot(aes(x=time,y=value,color=variable))+
geom_line(size=2)+
theme_classic()+
labs(x='time (yr)',y='number of individuals')
```

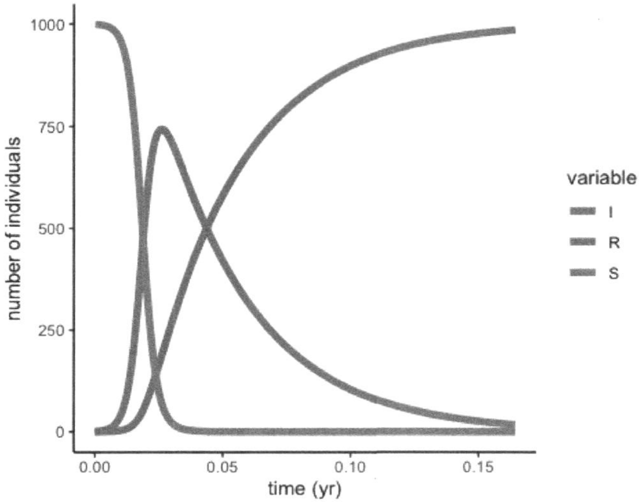

Figure 2.3 SIR model simulation

2.3 SEIR model

The standard deterministic SEIR model (30) has compartments for susceptible (S), exposed-not-infectious (E), infectious (I) and recovered (R). Neither this nor the SIR model account for PCR detectability. The compartmental transition equations are given by:

$$\frac{dS}{dt} = -\beta S \cdot I/N \tag{2.4}$$

$$\frac{dE}{dt} = \beta S \cdot I/N - \sigma E \tag{2.5}$$

$$\frac{dI}{dt} = \sigma * E - \gamma * I \tag{2.6}$$

$$\frac{dR}{dt} = \gamma I \tag{2.7}$$

```
closed.seir.model <- function (t, x, params) {
  ## first extract the state variables
  S <- x[1]
  E <- x[2]
  I <- x[3]
  R <- x[4]
  ## now extract the parameters
  beta <- params["beta"]
  gamma <- params["gamma"]
  sigma<- params["sigma"]
  N <- S+E+I+R
  ## now code the model equations
  dSdt <- -beta*S*I/N
  dEdt<-  beta*S*I/N - sigma*E
  dIdt <- sigma*E -gamma*I
  dRdt <- gamma*I
  ## combine results into a single vector
  dxdt <- c(dSdt,dEdt,dIdt,dRdt)
  ## return result as a list!
  list(dxdt)
}
```

To simulate the above model, we follow:

```
parms <- c(beta=400,gamma=365/13,sigma=50)

times <- seq(from=0,to=60/365,by=1/365/4)
xstart <- c(S=999,E=0,I=1,R=0)
ode(
  func=closed.seir.model,
  y=xstart,
  times=times,
  parms=parms
) %>%
  as.data.frame() -> out2
```

```
out2 %>%
gather(variable,value,-time) %>%
ggplot(aes(x=time,y=value,color=variable))+
geom_line(size=2)+
theme_classic()+
labs(x='time (yr)',y='number of individuals')
```

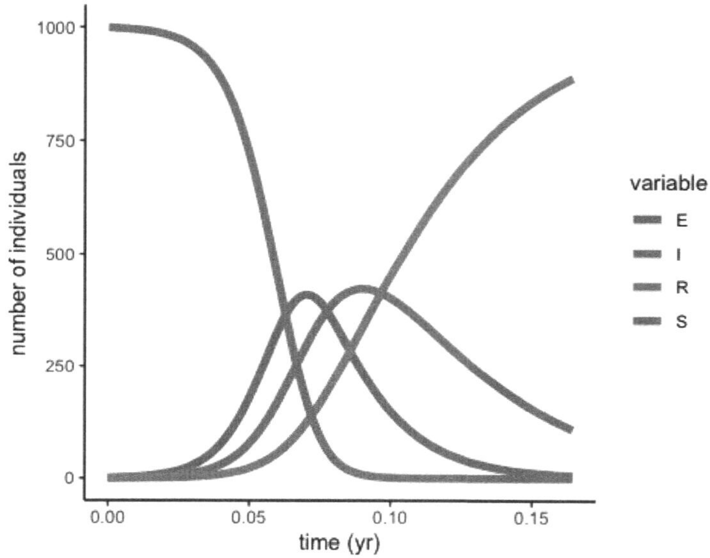

Figure 2.4 SEIR model simulation

2.4 A comparative appraisal of SIR and SEIR models

```
ggplot(data=out2, aes(x=I, y=R))+
 geom_path(arrow = arrow())+
 geom_point(data=out,aes(x=I, y=R))+
 labs(title="Thin SIR,thicker SEIR")
```

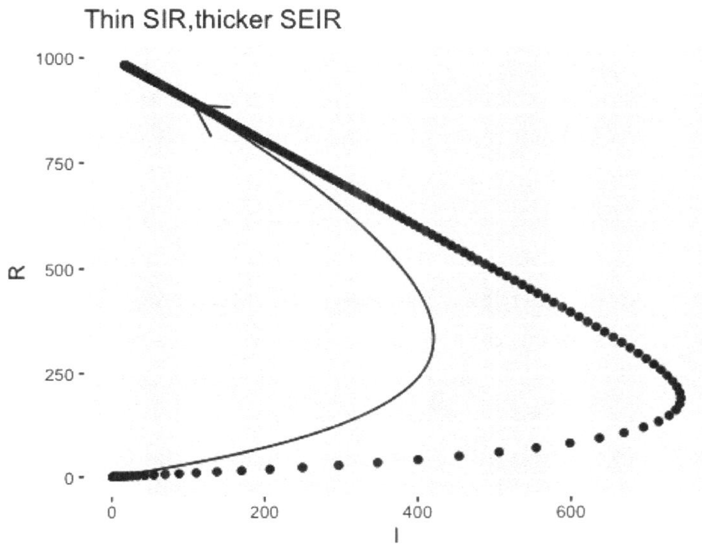

Figure 2.5 SIR- SEIR comparison

The comparison shows that a steady recovery is expected in both models, while in the SEIR model, the infection passes through a bigger surge (31).

2.5 Some applications of these classic Epidemiological models

- The SIR model was used to predict the spread of measles in the United States during the 1960s. The model showed that the measles vaccination program effectively reduced the number of measles cases (32).
- The SEIR model was used to study the spread of influenza during the 2009 H1N1 pandemic. The model showed that the pandemic could have been more severe without a vaccination program (33).

- The SEIRR model was being used to study the spread of COVID-19. The model informs public health policy decisions, such as when to implement lockdown measures. The SEEIRR (34) model can be regarded as a modified form of the SEIR model in which the exposed population has been split into (a) detectable E1 and (b) exposed noninfectious detectable E2. Similarly, the recovered population has been divided into (a) recovered-noninfectious detectable and (b) recovered noninfectious undetectable. This model has an edge over the preceding models as one correlates the Ct values of the RT-PCR tests from these additional compartments (E2/E1 and R2/R1). In the generalized SEEIRR model, the above relation is further generalized, assuming that two classes of exposed population (E1 and E2).

2.6 Ct value model as a Gaussian process

Let us introduce the daily probability of infection as π_t where infection on that day could result in a positive PCR test on the testing day. For a Gaussian process prior for a vector k, we can express: The equation, when sketched, leads to the following profile for a SEIR-based model:

$$\pi_t = \frac{1}{1 + exp(-k_t t)} \tag{2.8}$$

The equation 2.8, when analyzed, leads to the approach of π_t to 1 indicating inevitable occurrence of infection.

2.7 R number and the epidemiological models

> ⓘ Note
>
> The R number is also known as R-naught in social media. The R-naught value, or the reproduction number, indicates the rate of spread of a disease or infection among the population. It denotes the average number of people an infected person is likely to spread the disease.

A year ago, the term R number hardly made any sense to a layman. With the pandemic hanging around our necks, suddenly (like RT PCR), everyone is talking about R-number. If we assume the existence of a very crude model of an epidemic in which the infected population satisfies the discrete equation.

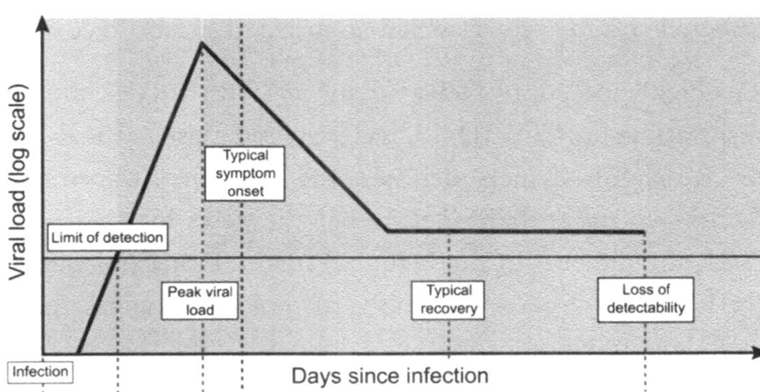

Figure 2.6 Time profile of viral load

The R number is a way of rating coronavirus or any disease's ability to spread. R can be approximately defined as the average number of people to whom a single infected person will transmit a virus. Measles has an R number of 15 in populations without immunity. That means, on average, one person will spread measles to 15 others. Coronavirus first identified in China's Wuhan (known officially as Sars-CoV-2) has a R number of 3. Among the different variants, while the alpha variant has R number of 5, the delta variant has an R-value close to 6-8.

The correlation of the model with the basic reproduction model can be performed by correlating the model parameters with the R number (for the simplest case, say, the SIR model):

$$R = \beta \cdot \gamma \tag{2.9}$$

The above relation expressed in equation reveals the identical ground truth that the primary reproductive number (R number) becomes a product of the rate at which a susceptible individual in contact with an infected person becomes infected and the rate at which an infected person recovers.

The highly infectious Delta variant of SARS-CoV-2, the virus responsible for COVID-19, has triggered a rise in the R-value or R-naught—which denotes the effective transmission factor—to more than one. As per the news byte on Aug 2, 2021, the director of the National Institute of Epidemiology (NIE) said, "A combination of epidemiological factors including infection growth rate, increasing number of deaths and hospital occupancy rate explain the risk." At that time, the national average of R-naught was 1.01, and the value was around 1.4 at the peak of the second wave in May, but it later declined to 0.7. While an increase in R-naught is worrying, many experts say a state/district cannot be "red-zoned" just because the R-value is rising. At least ten states in India had an R-value more than the national average of 1.01 at one point of time. According to NewByytes App, MP had the highest R-naught of 1.31, while HP, Nagaland, and Kerala have 1.30, 1.09, and 1.06, respectively. Both Delhi and Maharashtra had an R-value of 1.01 as well. However, the above stat is contradicted by MINT(same date) https://www.livemint.com/news/india/covid19-second-wave-still-not-over-r-value-up-in-8-states-warns-centre-11627990109891.html, according to whom Himachal Pradesh topped the list. The contradiction also points out the lack of trust in different news media and different methods of R-naught evaluation. Unfortunately, some scientists (e.g., IIMSC, Chennai, and Director NIE) were also involved in these contradictory statements.

2.8 Other Fine Structure Models of COVID Infection Dynamics

2.8.1 NGM method of expressing the reproductive number

The work by (35) showed a bistability-like phenomenon in the COVID outbreak for the first time. Their model calculates the basic reproduction number, R0, using the next-generation matrix method (36). The basic reproductive number R_0 is related to responses to both questions. Definitions of R_0 are often interpreted as the expected number of new infections created by a single (typical) infectious individual in a population that is otherwise completely uninfected.

$$R_0 = \frac{infections}{times \cdot infected}(duration\ of\ infection) \quad (2.10)$$

The RHS of equation (2.10) $\frac{infections}{times \cdot infected}$ is the expected number of people that one person will infect per unit time. When we multiply by the duration of infection, we get the expected number of people that one person will infect over the entire time during their disease period. If the R0 number is greater than 1, then—on average—more infected people replace themselves (increasing the infected population by more than 1) before recovery (which reduces the infected population by 1), and the disease grows. If this number is less than 1, on average, infected people do not replace themselves before they recover, and the disease gradually dies out.

$If(R_0 > 1)$ the disease grows

Else,

the disease remains steady

or dies out

2.8.2 The Matrix Model

The Matrix Model can be expressed by:

$$R = \frac{Infection \quad Rate}{Recovery \quad Rate} \tag{2.11}$$

$$R = FV.^{-1} \tag{2.12}$$

If infected classes are expressed by a vector Y,

$$Y(t+1) = RY(t) \tag{2.13}$$

$$Y(t) = R^t Y(0) \tag{2.14}$$

If express the equation using the eigenvector expression:

$$RY = \lambda Y \tag{2.15}$$

we have a simple expression for Y,

$$Y(t) = \lambda^t Y(0) \tag{2.16}$$

We can thus write down the general matrix equation, and then consider the $\rho(FV^{-1})$ *dominant eigenvalue* λ so that we connect the matrix R with R_0

$$R_0 = \lambda = \rho(FV^{-1}) \tag{2.17}$$

2.9 Parameters of the model

Table 2.2 Parameters of the model

Parameters	Meaning	Values
Π	Rate of Population Increase	Varies
$\frac{1}{\mu}$	Av. Life. Expectancy.	Varies
β	Transmission Rate	0-200 per day
r	Lock Down Efficiency	0-1
$\frac{1}{\gamma}$	Covid Incubation Period	1-14 Days
1	Av. Life. Expectancy	0-1
η	Av. Life. Expectancy	Varies
δ	Hospital Death Rate	Varies
τ_1	Recovery Rate symptomatic	0-1 per day
$\frac{1}{\psi}$	Lock Down Period	Varies
τ_2	Recovery Rate hospitalized	Varies

2.10 Agent-based models for COVID-19

2.10.1 Idea of an Agent-Based Model

Agent-based models are computer simulations that study interactions between people, things, places, and time. These models are built from the bottom up, meaning that individual agents are created and assigned to specific attributes. The agents are then programmed to behave and interact with each other and the environment in specific ways. These interactions can produce emergent effects, which are not directly caused by any individual agent but rather by the collective behavior of the agents.

Agent-based models differ from traditional, regression-based methods in that they allow for the exploration of complex systems that display non-independence of individuals and feedback loops in causal mechanisms. This means that agent-based models can be used to study systems where the behavior of one individual can affect the behavior of other individuals and where the effects of a particular action can depend on the order in which it is taken.

Agent-based models are also not limited to observed data. This means they can be used to model counterfactual or hypothetical scenarios that may be impossible or unethical to conduct in the real world. For example, an agent-based model could be used to simulate the spread of a disease under different vaccination rates or social distancing policies.

However, agent-based models have their limitations. One significant challenge is obtaining reliable data parameters required to construct the models, which are often scarce or hard to find in the literature. Additionally, assessing the validity of these models can be challenging, particularly when they involve unobserved or complex associations that need more direct empirical evidence.

2.11 Analytical approaches to the COVID-19 diagnosis

No doubt, the COVID-19 pressure has taught the 'laymen' many academic terms that otherwise were the forte of erudite academics. The term RT-PCR (37) is now familiar to a wide section of the population who have never heard about it before.

RT-PCR is a class of Nucleic acid amplification tests (NAATs). These tests are the most common and accurate way to diagnose COVID-19. They work by amplifying the virus's genetic material to detect it even in small amounts. NAATs include real-time *reverse transcription polymerase chain reaction (RT-PCR), loop-mediated isothermal amplification (LAMP), and transcription-mediated amplification (TMA).

Antigen tests: These tests detect the presence of viral antigens, which are proteins found on the virus's surface. Antigen tests are less sensitive than NAATs but can screen large numbers of people quickly.

Serological tests: These tests detect the presence of antibodies to the virus. Antibodies are proteins that the body produces in response to an infection. Serological tests can determine if someone has been infected with the virus in the past, but they cannot be used to diagnose an active infection.

Imaging tests: These tests can be used to look for signs of COVID-19 in the lungs. Imaging tests include chest X-rays and computed tomography (CT) scans. However, imaging tests are not as sensitive as NAATs or antigen tests and cannot be used to diagnose COVID-19 definitively. Many other conditions can mimic COVID-19 lung changes. AI can play a significant role in the screening of images and making a reasonable diagnosis

2.11.1 RT PCR is the gold standard

> ⓘ Important
>
> Real-time reverse transcription polymerase chain reaction (RT-PCR) is the gold standard for diagnosing COVID-19. It is a highly sensitive and specific test that can detect the virus's genetic material, even in small amounts.

2.11.2 Limitations of RT-PCR

False negatives: RT-PCR tests can sometimes yield false negative results, indicating that a person does not have COVID-19 when, in reality, they are infected. This may occur if testing is done too early in the course of the infection, when the virus's genetic material is not yet present at detectable levels. False negatives can also result from improper sample collection or errors in the testing process.

False positives: RT-PCR tests can also yield false positive results, indicating that a person has COVID-19 when they do not. This may occur if the person has been exposed to a virus with genetic material similar to SARS-CoV-2, such as certain strains of the common cold virus. False positives can also result from contamination during the testing process.

Inability to detect past infections: RT-PCR tests can only detect the presence of the virus's genetic material in the present. They cannot detect past infections, which is essential for understanding the development and spread of the virus.

2.11.3 RT-PCR principle

In the first step, there is no amplification, only reverse transcription of mRNA to cDNA. The equation that follows is

$$[cDNA] = [RNA] \cdot \eta_{RT} \tag{2.18}$$

Efficiency η_{RT} is measured as the percentage of RNA transcribed into cDNA.Typically, the efficiency can fluctuate from 5%–90%. The PCR product can be expressed by the equation:

$$NC = [cDNA] \cdot (\eta_{PCR} + 1)^{n_{cycle}} \tag{2.19}$$

η_{PCR} being the efficiency of the PCR.In competitive RT-PCR, a dilution series of the standard RNA is co-amplified with equal amounts of total RNA (and, therefore, equal amounts of the native gene). Competitive RT-PCR is the most common approach to quantitative RT-PCR. Conventionally, the Ct value performs the presence or absence of an RNA virus template, indicating the threshold n_{cycle} at which the fluorescence generated within a reaction crosses the fluorescence threshold, a fluorescent signal significantly above the background fluorescence. At the threshold cycle, a detectable amount of amplicon product has been generated during the early exponential phase of the reaction. The threshold cycle is inversely proportional to the original relative expression level of the gene of interest. [1] One should keep in mind that a substantial proportion of COVID-19-positive cases with cycle threshold (Ct) values more than or equal to 31 were subsequently tested negative for SARS-CoV-2 RNA within 7 days of initial detection of the viral load.

2.12 CRISPR-based tests for COVID-19

For CRISPR-based tests, we need to use gRNA.

> ⓘ Note
>
> gRNA stands for guide RNA. A short synthetic RNA sequence directs CRISPR-Cas enzymes to specific DNA or RNA targets.

> ⓘ Note
>
> CRISPR-Cas enzymes are naturally occurring proteins that can be programmed to cut DNA or RNA at specific sequences.

CRISPR-Cas enzymes can be utilized to diagnose diseases by identifying specific DNA or RNA sequences in a sample. This technology has applications in diagnosing genetic disorders, infectious diseases, and cancers. For COVID-19,

---

[1] The RT PCR test usually declares someone as COVID-negative if the Ct value $\geq$ 31.

CRISPR-based tests work by employing CRISPR-Cas enzymes to detect the presence of SARS-CoV-2 RNA in a sample. CRISPR-Cas enzymes are naturally occurring proteins that can be programmed to recognize and cut specific DNA or RNA sequences.

To develop a CRISPR-based test for COVID-19, scientists first identify a unique sequence of SARS-CoV-2 RNA. Then, they design a guide RNA (gRNA) molecule that is complementary to this sequence. The gRNA molecule leads the CRISPR-Cas enzyme to the target sequence of SARS-CoV-2 RNA.

If SARS-CoV-2 RNA is present in the sample, the CRISPR-Cas enzyme will cut it. This cleavage event can be detected using various methods, such as fluorescence or colorimetric detection.

CRISPR-based tests for COVID-19 are highly sensitive and specific. This means that they can detect even small amounts of SARS-CoV-2 RNA in a sample and are unlikely to produce false positive results.

> ⓘ Note
>
> For example, gRNA sequence 5'-GGTTGGGTGC GGAGGTATGC-3' is complementary to a unique sequence of RNA in the Delta variant of SARS-CoV-2.

The steps to be followed for COVID-19 detection are described as follows:

A sample of saliva or nasal swab is collected from the patient. The RNA is extracted from the sample. The RNA is mixed with a CRISPR-Cas enzyme and a gRNA molecule complementary to a unique sequence of SARS-CoV-2 RNA. If SARS-CoV-2 RNA is present in the sample, the CRISPR-Cas enzyme will cut it. The cleavage event is detected using a fluorescence or colourimetric detection method. If the cleavage event is detected, the patient is positive for COVID-19. If the cleavage event is undetected, the patient is negative for COVID-19.

3.
Being a Detective: Lab Leak Versus Zoonosis

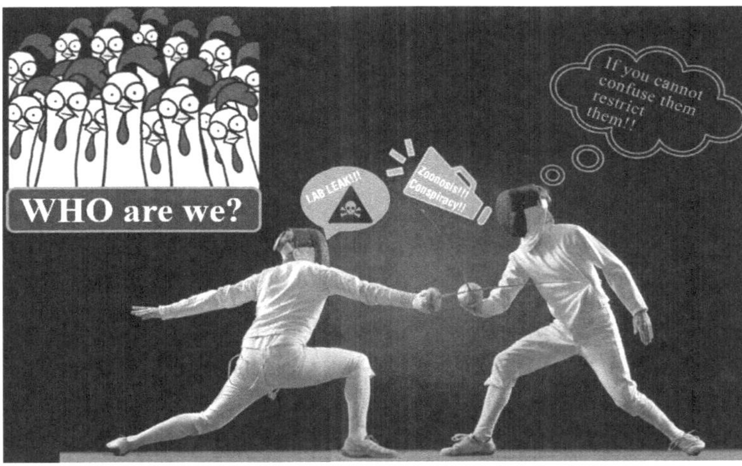
WHO are we?
LAB LEAK!!!
Zoonosis!!!
Conspiracy!!
If you cannot confuse them restrict them!!

Figure 3.1 The debate around the origin of COVID 19

According to theworldometers (https://www. worldometers. info/coronavirus/) the overall world scenario of the corona virus cases till 31st Aug 2021 can be summarized as follows:

Table 3.1 A brief inventory of the epidemics

Cases	**Deaths**	**Recovered**	**%recovery**	**%death**
217987071	4525210	194893916	89.40618	2.075908

The families of those who have lost lives as well as those who want to prevent such pandemics are very keen to know about the origin of the disease.

3.1 Hypothesis I

The popular hypotheses so far have been lab-leak or inadvertent infection from Wuhan Institute of Virology where gain-of-function studies were being carried out on the viruses.

3.2 Hypothesis II

Zoonoses originated from the Wuhan seafood market. However, China's vehement reluctance to share information has thwarted WHO's efforts so far. To add to the woes many scientists and reporters have pointed out that History provides us with multiple instances of inadvertent release of pathogenic agents that have resulted in loss of lives.

Evidence in favour of zoonosis: Genomic analysis shows similarities between SARS-CoV-2 and other coronaviruses found in bats (e.g., RaTG13, with ~96% genomic similarity) and pangolins (~91% similarity). The virus is thought to have acquired the ability to infect humans via mutations in the spike protein.

3.3 Some old stories

3.3.1 The Birmingham leak

Do we not remember the most controversial spread of variola/smallpox virus in 1978 from the smallpox laboratory in Birmingham University Medical School, resulting in an outbreak just before smallpox was about to be declared eradicated by the WHO (38). Not only did it result in the death of infected Mrs. Janet Parker, the medical photographer working there but, also led to the untimely loss of the distraught laboratory head, a renowned scientist, Prof Henry Bedson (https://www.bbc.com/news/uk-england-birmingham-45101091).

3.3.2 The NIH leak

In 2014, vials of virus stocks were discovered inside a cardboard box in a refrigerator at the National Institutes of Health (NIH) campus in Bethesda during routine inventory checks (39).

3.3.3 The anthrax scares in the city of Sverdlovsk

Another disaster was born during the Cold War, uncovered to the world after 13 years. The guilty pathogen Bacillus anthracis (40) was used by the Soviet Union. In the year 1979, the city of Sverdlovsk in erstwhile USSR recorded an unusual outbreak of gastrointestinal and cutaneous anthrax which the iron curtain nation quickly covered up claiming tainted meat consumption (striking similarity with the Wuhan episode is notable). Russian President, Boris Yeltsin had to accept the presence of a biological weapons unit as the likely source of Bacillus spores and allowed a team of scientists led by Prof. Matthew Meselson to investigate.

3.3.4 A Bio-terror activity in Calcutta

A zamindar from Pakur was murdered by pricking a Yersinia pestis laced needle in 1933 by his own stepbrother. Dr Nalini Ranjan Sengupta, a famous physician then had prescribed a blood culture which led to the discovery of the pathogen and subsequent investigation by Kolkata police on the smuggling of the bacteria from Haffkine Institute for Training, Research and Testing, Mumbai resulted in the prosecution of the culprits (https://scroll.in/article/868697/prick-of-death-how-the-calcutta-police-solved-one-of-indias-first-cases-of-biocrime-85-years-ago)

The origin of SARS-CoV-2 continues to be an area of scientific and geopolitical debate, and any new findings could refine or shift the current understanding.

3.4 Timeline of the COVID outbreak

It may be noted that WHO declared a PHEIC (Public Health Emergency of International Concern) alert after some hesitations in spite of a few revealing publications appearing at that time (41).

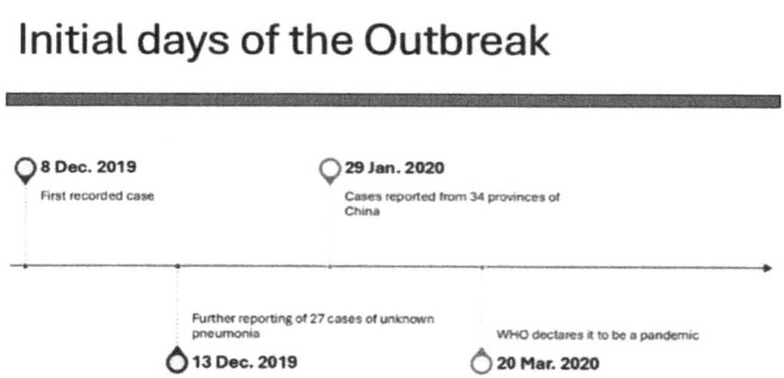

Figure 3.2 Timeline of the initial outbreak of the pandemic

3.5 PubMed literature on COVID

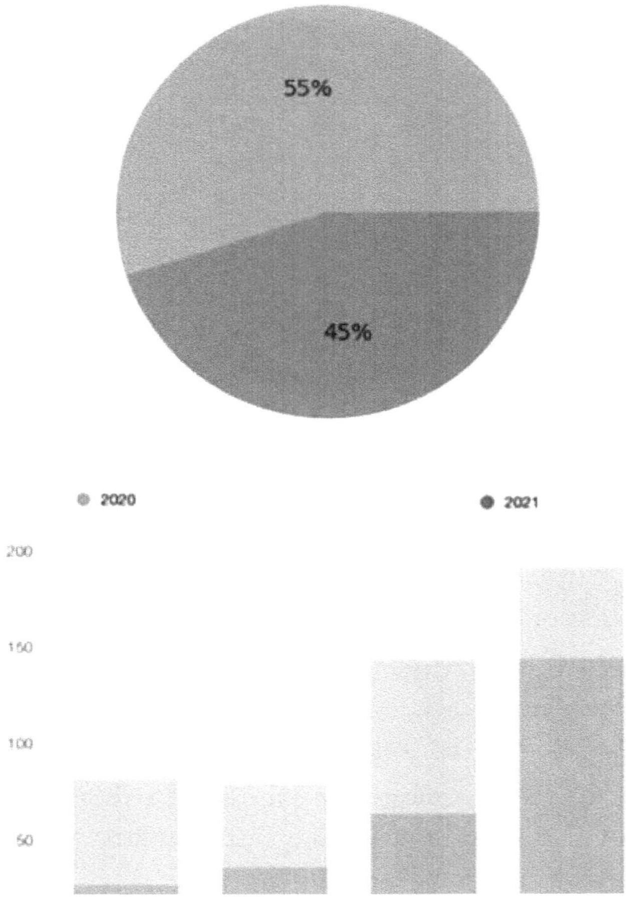

Figure 3.3 PubMed citation on Covid

3.6 The spike protein

The S protein is a highly glycosylated and large type I transmembrane fusion protein that gives rise to the spike-shaped protrusions found on the surface of the coronavirus. A few pieces of information may be helpful at this stage concerning the spike (S) protein:

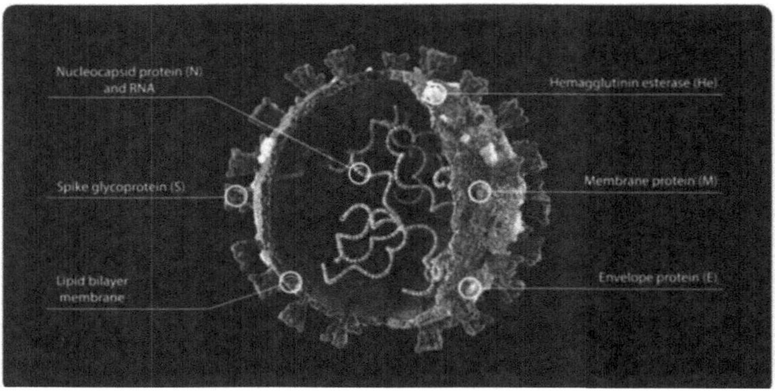

Figure 3.4 Spike Protein

- The SARS-CoV-2 S protein has a full size of 1,273 amino acids, longer than that of SARS-CoV (1,255 amino acids)
- bat-originated SARSr-CoVs (1,245–1,269 amino acids).
- In the receptor-binding domain (RBD) of the S protein, the amino acid similarity between SARS-CoV-2 and SARS-CoV is 73%.
- Another specific genomic feature of SARS-CoV-2 is the insertion of four amino acid residues (PRRA) i.e., proline-arginine-arginine-alanine at the junction of subunits S1 and S2 of the S protein.
- Proline is established as a potent breaker of both alpha-helical and beta-sheet structures in soluble (globular) proteins.

- This insertion generates a polybasic cleavage site (RRAR), which enables effective cleavage by furin and other proteases.
- Because furin proteases are abundant in the respiratory tract, it is possible that SARS-CoV-2 S glycoprotein is cleaved upon exit from epithelial cells and consequently can efficiently infect other cells.
- In contrast, the highly related bat CoV RaTG-13 does not have the furin cleavage site.
- Such an S1–S2 cleavage site is not observed in all related viruses belonging to the subgenus Sarbecovirus, except for a similar three amino acid insertion (PAA) in RmYN02, a bat-derived coronavirus newly reported from Rhinolophus malayanus in China.

3.7 Mutations in S protein and the origin of variants

The glycosylated S protein has two subunits near its N and C terminal (the two locations which are normally marked as the beginning and end of a peptide chain - and assemble of such peptides constitute the protein).

- The N-terminal S1
- The C-terminal S2

It is the S1 region that would bind to the host receptor and undergo many mutations whereas the S2 region remains more or less conserved. S proteins can be regarded as primary agents for interaction with host cells as without the S, the SARS-COV-2 would not be able to interact with any host cell. In addition to its role in penetrating host cells, the S protein is also responsible for inducing NAbs (neutralizing antibodies). To elicit antiviral activity NAbs would bind to the surface epitopes of viral particles to prevent their entry into the cells. The Variants have been classified as described in the table accompanying 3.12

The NCBI Datasets Project has developed virus-specific genome and protein datasets, initially limited to the Coronaviridae (NCBI Taxonomy ID: 11118) family of viruses, in response to the COVID-19 pandemic. Viral genome data is currently limited to all Coronaviridae (Taxonomy ID: 11118) including SARS-CoV-2 (SARS2, Taxonomy ID: 2697049). Viral protein data is currently limited to SARS-CoV-2 (SARS2) only.

3.8 Covid Variants and the root of the debate

The first SARS-CoV-2 genome sequence information was made available to the scientific community on the 10th of January 2020. The GISAID(https://gisaid.org/) and NCBI databases (https://www.ncbi.nlm.nih.gov/sars-cov-2) house around 13,758,184 and 6,416,687 wgs of SARS-CoV2, respectively (as on 3rd November, 2022). The GISAID and Pangolin databases assign a newly sequenced SARS-CoV-2 genome to a clade and a lineage. Knowing the genome and its dynamics is crucial for the scientific community for several reasons.

3.9 Importance of Understanding the Viral Genome

The viral genome contains the blueprint of the viral life cycle. It encodes information that is translated into multiple proteins, which are responsible for the virus's activities. Any changes in the genome sequence can lead to alterations in the proteins, impacting the virus's behavior and characteristics. Monitoring such changes is essential for global tracking of SARS-CoV-2, pandemic management, and even in designing RT-PCR tests.

3.10 Factors Enabling Worldwide Dissemination of Viral Sequence Information

The successful dissemination of viral sequence information worldwide was facilitated by three crucial elements:

1. **Advances in Sequencing Technology:** The dip in sequencing time and costs over the past decade due to advancements in next-generation sequencing technology.
2. **Data Sharing:** Despite challenges in data sharing, the pandemic has encouraged better data sharing among countries and organizations. The GISAID database played a significant role in providing a platform for swift and free access to epidemic and pandemic virus data.
3. **GISAID Database:** The Global Initiative on Sharing All Influenza Data (GISAID) database became a reliable platform for researchers and public health officials, fostering private-public partnerships. It allows sharing of sequence data and related clinical and epidemiological information, aiding the understanding of viral evolution and spread.

3.11 Understanding the SARS-CoV-2 Genome Specifics

The SARS-CoV-2 genome consists of 29,811 nucleotides, encoding 29 proteins responsible for the virus's functions. These proteins include non-structural proteins (NSP1-16), accessory proteins (3a, 3b, 6, 7a, 7b, 8, 9b, 9c & 10), and structural proteins (Spike, Membrane, Envelope, and Nucleocapsid). Genetic variants or mutations can lead to changes in these proteins, affecting the virus's behavior and its interactions with the host.

3.12 Variant Classification Scheme

The US government SARS-CoV-2 Interagency Group (SIG) developed a variant classification scheme, including Variants of Interest (VOI), Variants of Concern (VOC), and Variants of High Consequence (VOHC). These classifications are based on the impact of mutations on the virus's activity, transmissibility, and disease severity as described in the accompanying table 3.2.

Table 3.2 A brief description of mutations and their impacts

Category Definition	Examples	Key Mutations	Impact
Variants of Interest (VOI) Variants with genetic changes that may affect virus characteristics and are identified as causing community spread.	- Mu (B.1.621) - Lambda (C.37)	- Mutations in spike protein (e.g., E484K)	Potential for reduced neutralization by antibodies or increased transmissibility, under investigation.
Variants of Concern (VOC) Variants that show increased transmissibility, disease severity, or reduced effectiveness of treatments/vaccines.	- Alpha (B.1.1.7) - Beta (B.1.351) - Gamma (P.1) - Delta (B.1.617.2) - Omicron (BA.1, BA.2, XBB, etc.)	- N501Y (Alpha, Beta, Gamma) - E484K (Beta, Gamma) - L452R (Delta) - S:Omicron-specific mutations (Omicron)	Increased transmissibility, immune escape, higher risk of reinfection, reduced vaccine effectiveness.
Variants of High Consequence (VOHC) Variants with clear evidence of significantly reduced effectiveness of preventive or therapeutic measures.	None identified to date	N/A	Hypothetical category reserved for future variants that cause a major public health crisis.

3.13 Clade and Lineage Classification

Different groups and initiatives have proposed classification schemes based on viral mutations and lineage information. The GISAID initiative defined major variant groups as clades based on differences from the reference Wuhan genome. The NextStrain project followed a clade classification based on the year and frequency of variants. Professors Rambaut and Plybus introduced the 'lineage' or 'Pango lineage' system, considering mutations affecting viral activity and spread.

3.14 The Delta Variant

The Delta variant (Pango lineage B.1.617.2, clade GK, Nextstrain clade 21A/S:478K) has garnered attention for its increased transmissibility and potential resistance to some treatments. It is classified as a Variant of Concern (VOC) due to its impact on transmission and vaccine efficacy.

3.15 The Lab Origin Debate

The origin of the polybasic proteolytic cleavage site found in SARS-CoV-2 is a subject of debate between natural selection (zoonosis) and lab-origin theories. The site's natural evolution or artificial manipulation in a laboratory remains contentious.

3.16 The vanity fair report (August 2021)

While the media was all busy in reporting the Afghan horror, there was a major revelation in the US media regarding the origin of COVID-19. Some key features of this declassification report are: - There is a possibility that the virus leaked from a laboratory in Wuhan, China - This is in contrast with the consensus till July of 2021 that the virus evolved out of natural evolution and the lab-leak hypothesis could be dismissed as a conspiracy theory - But intelligence agencies split over the likeliest explanation for how it leaped to humans, with the National Intelligence Council and four other agencies favoring a natural origin, one favoring a lab leak of some kind, and three undecided.

https://www.vanityfair.com/news/2021/08/bidens-covid-19-origins-report-leaves-the-lab-leak-on-the-table

3.17 Broader perspective

3.17.1 Encouraging the Gain of function (GOF) research

Gain-of-function research refers to the serial passaging of microorganisms to increase their transmissibility, virulence, immunogenicity, and host tropism by applying selective pressure to a culture. The early microbiologist working on Cholera knew that the strain virulence increases with animal passage (rabbit ileal loop,(42)).

3.17.2 Fauci-Rand Paul debate

On July 15, 2021, Rand Paul and Fauci debated the possible role of NIH in the GOF. While Fauci denied the allegation that the NIH had been funding the Wuhan Virology project on GOF, this has become a subject of intense debate between Democrats and Republicans, Democrats support the stand taken by Fauci. As early as 2010 there was a WHO guidance document for DURC (dual use research of concern), indicating the potential military use of biology and biomedical research. The debate ultimately headed towards the gain of function (GOF) research. Any organism can acquire a new ability or property, or "gain" a "function". This can happen through natural selection or a researcher's experiments. In research, many different types of experiments generate functions, and some pose certain safety and security concerns. The issue of gain of function research however came under scrutiny in 2012, when a team of Japanese scientists in the US published a paper that helped show how the avian flu H5N1 may have been transmitted to humans. There was however a strong solicitation from some quarters of US scientists on the importance of GOF (gain of function) research in drug and vaccine discovery etc. The article (43) may be contextual. There was indeed a GOF project in the Wuhan lab and the project was indeed funded by NIH. So if there is a conspiracy at all; the same was hatched collaboratively.

3.17.3 A detail of the collaboration

The article describes the collaboration between Ralph Baric from the University of North Carolina and Shi from China. They started collaborating on a GOF project. Baric used a reverse genetic approach in which he could induct new functions into a virus. For example, he wanted to take the spike gene from SHCO14 and move it to a genetic copy of a SARS virus which he already has in his lab. His objective was to enable the spike of SHCO14 in human cells. While this was happening from 2013 onwards, before 2015 the NIH announced that it would halt granting the GOF research. After an initial halt, Baric could continue the research by convincing the NIH panel that he could continue the studies at minimal risk. NIH funded $600000 between 2014 to 2019 and till now has refused to release a copy of the grant. With the help of Fauci (who denied any involvement in GOF), the project was continued in the Wuhan lab.

3.17.4 The origin of COVID-19 will remain a Schrodinger cat

It appears that like the unverified death of Netaji Bose by a plane crash, the origin of COVID-19 will remain elusive as the most important and powerful nations collaborated in GOF research though whether this was an outcome of such GOF or a result of a spontaneous mutation (which many scientists particularly those based in China and US vouch for) would remain elusive for years to come.

3.18 Vaccination

The vaccination program posed a challenge comparable to the Manhattan Project. Like the Manhattan Project, the collective efforts of scientists from different labs won the war. This war is not only against the virus, but against the anti-vaxxers, the naysayers, and the scientists who thought that vaccine should be provided only after a sufficiently long testing time. Some of them were technically correct as it follows the standard medical protocol to subject this kind of new vaccine under the strictest possible scrutiny. But we in the process learned the lesson that sometimes the instincts we perceive take precedence over well devoted protocols.

If we do not survive, there will be no takers for the protocol.

Here is a summary of all the vaccines used till now.

Table 3.3 Vaccines approved and used during the pandemic

Vaccine Name	Technology	Efficacy	Safety Profile	Country of Manufac-ture
Pfizer-BioNTech (Comirnaty)	mRNA	~95% against symptomatic infection (pre-Omicron); reduced efficacy against Omicron but effective for severe disease	Mild side effects (fever, fatigue, headache); rare myocarditis in young males; robust safety data overall	USA, Germany
Moderna (Spikevax)	mRNA	~94.1% against symptomatic infection (pre-Omicron); strong efficacy against severe disease	Similar to Pfizer; mild to moderate side effects; rare myocarditis reported	USA
AstraZeneca (Vaxzevria/ Covishield)	Viral vector (adenovirus)	~70% overall efficacy; ~76-85% against severe disease	Common: fever, fatigue, injection site pain; rare blood clotting (VITT) linked with low platelets	UK, India (Covishield by Serum Institute)
Johnson & Johnson (Janssen)	Viral vector (adenovirus)	~66% against moderate-to-severe infection globally; ~85% against severe disease	Common side effects; rare cases of thrombosis with thrombocytopenia (VITT)	USA
Sinovac (CoronaVac)	Inactivated virus	~50-84% efficacy against symptomatic infection; effective against severe disease	Mild to moderate side effects; generally safe in broad populations	China
Sinopharm (BBIBP-CorV)	Inactivated virus	~79% efficacy against symptomatic infection (based on trials); effective against severe disease	Similar safety profile to Sinovac; generally well-tolerated	China

Vaccine Name	Technology	Efficacy	Safety Profile	Country of Manufacture
Covaxin (Bharat Biotech)	Inactivated virus	~78% efficacy against symptomatic infection; effective against severe disease	Mild to moderate side effects; no major safety concerns reported	India
Sputnik V	Viral vector (adenovirus)	~91.6% efficacy against symptomatic infection; strong protection against severe disease	Mild to moderate side effects; concerns over lack of transparency in safety data	Russia
Novavax (Nuvaxovid/ Covovax)	Protein subunit	~89-90% efficacy against symptomatic infection (pre-Omicron); high efficacy against severe disease	Mild side effects; good tolerability profile	USA, India (Covovax by Serum Institute)
CanSinoBIO (Convidecia)	Viral vector (adenovirus)	~65.7% efficacy against symptomatic infection; ~90% against severe disease	Similar to other adenovirus vaccines; generally mild side effects	China

The trend line for such global usage of vaccines is depicted below.

The pandemic has generated such large interest in scientific research that starting from theoretical physicists to quantum chemists, everyone has participated in the COVID research. While the medical fraternity was primarily bogged down by the scale of the clinical crisis, lack of definitive therapy, inadequate supply of oxygen, vaccine, and other management issues, there were many dedicated molecular biology virology and bioinformatics labs that wanted to crack the lethal viral transmission and vaccine or drug-related remedies of the same.

3.19 Country wise snapshot

Let us first look into the global population:

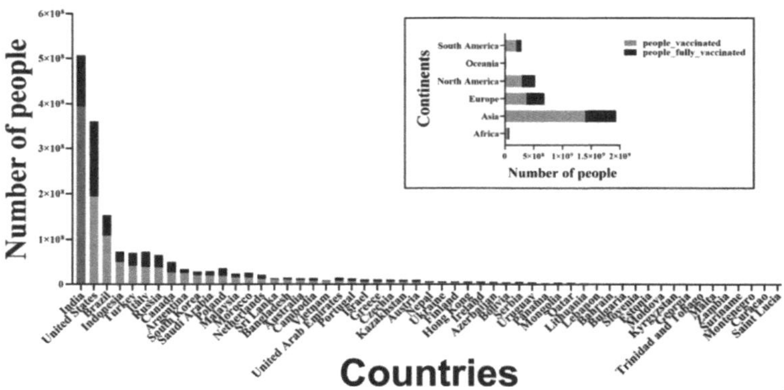

Figure .3.5 Country-wise vaccinated population

The Figure 3.5shows that India tops the list of the population who have got at least one vaccination. Even for the population doubly vaccinated India comes second to the US. If we normalize the statistical picture with vaccinated per 100, we get a completely different picture in Fig 3.6:

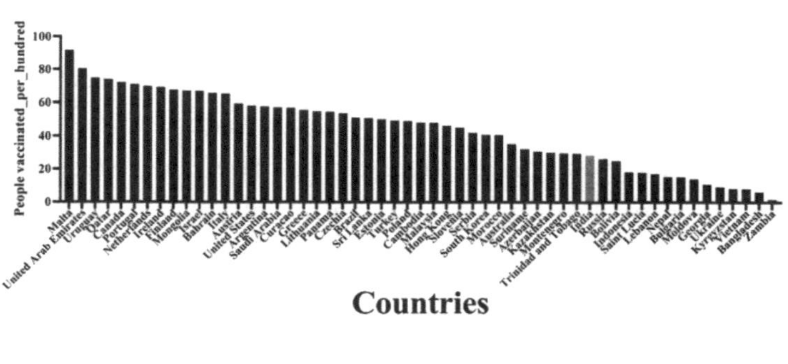

Figure 3.6 Country-wise vaccinated population (normalized per 100)

The normalized brings India to the bottom of the list (because of its huge population). The politics of vaccination starts from here. If we describe the figure 3.5 it will glorify India on the other hand if we only show figure 3.6 it will throw a poor light on the COVID management in India.

3.20 Warning Bells in the US and China

Very recently, the United States was in the midst of a new wave related to Omicron variants BA.2 and BA.2.12.1 with over 90,000 confirmed new cases a day and a 20% increase in hospitalizations.

Fortunately, the large spike of this variant with a high degree of infectivity has now subsided. People are however worried about the millions of infections in China. The Indian government. has also been alarmed and advised its people to take proper precautions in crowded places. However, there is a section of the media who are spreading panic among the common masses.

3.21 Masks politics

Any write-up on COVID -19 will remain incomplete unless we refer to the lifestyle changes it has caused all over the world. Starting from elbow touching instead of handshakes, and adapting to online classrooms and offices, the compulsion of mask-wearing in public places has created unrest in the western world (including the US). A US media report (July 29, 2021) details the tussle between a Republican leader (Kelvin McCarthy) and the ruling Democratic party (and the Center for Disease [CDC] Prevention) regarding a compulsory mask mandate. The allegation was that the latest regulation is based on data from India. The mandate from the CDC is a reversal of the May 2021 mandate that mask-wearing can be relaxed for fully vaccinated people. It may be noted that the dominance of delta variants might have changed the CDC's stand. The data from the CDC studies indicated that there was no significant difference between the virus load among infected and uninfected people. The reference to Indian Data was therefore a *racially charged political statement* from the republicans. The most important pro-mask mandate may have stemmed from the outbreak reports from Australia and China. A report published on July 30 ,2021 says "More than a year and a half after the coronavirus was first detected in China — followed by the world's first big wave of COVID-19 — the country is again battling to stem the spread of new cases attributed to the more infectious delta variant of the virus.", During the recurrence, fifteen Chinese cities had been affected. The rapid rate at which the Coronavirus originated in China and then got mutated in India with a significant increase in the R number was startling as well as mysterious

3.22 Happiness engineers versus the survey-based economics of COVID

The papers (Gans, 2020a, 2020b; Maxmen, 2021; Moosa, 2021),(Inoue, Murase and Todo, 2021; Kazemian, Fuller and Algara, 2021) provide some details of the economic impact of the COVID. The Mckinsey survey has revealed the public sentiment on COVID management. Most of the people (surveyed all across the globe) think that there would be a recurring impact on health and there would be slower near-term growth and delayed recovery. Notably, the number of people believing in the status quo remains somewhat increasing from 14% to 19%. In other words, "happiness engineering" fails despite the best possible narrative-building efforts by the surveyors.

3.23 Xmas 2022

While we almost forgot about the covid three things re-emerged that shook the world: (a) The twitter (X) files of COVID as exposed by Elon Musk (b) An explosion of infection in China (c) A reappearance of a covid variant strain in the US.

3.23.1 The Twitter (X) files of COVID

Let us consider the Twitter handle *David Zweig.* on Dec 26, 2022. The handle reveals a thread entitled "HOW TWITTER RIGGED THE COVID DEBATE". Twitter used the following protocol for the sensor:

> ⚠ Warning
>
> – By censoring info that was true but inconvenient to U.S. govt. policy – By discrediting doctors and other experts who disagreed – By suppressing ordinary users, including some sharing the CDC's *own data*

The next in the thread is:

> ⚠ Warning
>
> Twitter's secret blacklists - the company functioned as a kind of subsidiary of the FBI; rewrote the platform's rules to accommodate their political desires.

The most striking event is that both Trump and Biden administrations got involved in this coverup operation.

> ⚠ Warning
>
> Internal files showed that both the Trump and Biden administrations directly pressed Twitter(X) executives to moderate the platform's pandemic content according to their wishes.

The Biden-specific part of the expose was dedicated to the anti-vaxers.

> ⚠ Warning
>
> When the Biden admin took over, one of their first meeting requests with Twitter (X) executives was on Covid. The focus was on "anti-vaxxer accounts." Especially that of Alex Berenson.

3.23.2 Mutants versus variants

Viruses are constantly evolving and changing. Every time a virus replicates (makes copies of itself), there is the potential for there to be changes in its structure. Each of these changes is a "mutation." A virus with one or more mutations is called a "variant" of the original virus. If variants are expressed by a set $V \in V_1, V_2, .., V_N$ and mutations are expressed by a set M=$V \in M_1, M_2, .., M_K$ we may express:

$$V_i \cup Mi \in M \tag{3.1}$$

3.24 Side effects of Pfizer vaccine

As per the X handle @ ackStr42679640 Pfizer quiet press release on Paxlovid October 13, 2023, notes increased risk of myocarditis and pericarditis from Covid jabs with the highest prevalence in males 12 through 17.

In a press release published on 22nd August 2024, Pfizer has stated that "Myocarditis (inflammation of the heart muscle) and pericarditis (inflammation of the lining outside the heart) have occurred in some people who have received mRNA COVID-19 vaccines, including COMIRNATY and Pfizer-BioNTech COVID-19 vaccines. Myocarditis and pericarditis following COMIRNATY have occurred most commonly in adolescent males 12 through 17 years of age. In most of these individuals, symptoms began within a few days following vaccination. The chance of having this occur is very low. You should seek medical attention right away if you or your child have any of the following symptoms after receiving the vaccine, particularly during the 2 weeks after receiving a dose of the vaccine:

- Chest pain
- Shortness of breath
- Feelings of having a fast-beating, fluttering, or pounding heart
- No numbers have been mentioned, but the updated COVID-19 vaccine, tailored to the KP.2 strain of the SARS-CoV-2 Omicron JN.1 lineage has been approved by US FDA for individuals 6 months of age and older

- A number of Key Opinion Leaders in India had openly advocated the usage of this vaccine in India, but it was not approved by DCGI.

4.
Covid Controversies and the Future of Epidemics Management

The COVID-19 pandemic has generated several controversies and debates, some of which include:

- **Response of government and health organizations:** There has been criticism of the slow response of some governments and health organizations in addressing the COVID-19 pandemic, particularly regarding the availability of personal protective equipment (PPE) and implementing measures such as lockdowns and physical distancing.
- **Misinformation and conspiracy theories:** The pandemic has also been marked by the spread of misinformation and conspiracy theories, which has caused confusion and fear among the public. The infodemic was perhaps bigger than the pandemic itself. Some of these theories include false claims about the origins of the virus, the effectiveness of certain treatments, and the safety of vaccines.
- **Disparities in access to healthcare:** The COVID-19 pandemic has revealed and exacerbated existing disparities in access to healthcare, particularly among marginalized communities. There have been reports of racial and ethnic minority groups being disproportionately affected by the pandemic and of

limited access to testing and treatment in low-income communities.

- **Economic impact and government support:** The COVID-19 pandemic has devastated the global economy, leading to widespread job losses and financial insecurity. Governments around the world have implemented various measures to support workers and businesses. However, these measures have also been the subject of debate and criticism, particularly with regard to their effectiveness and distribution.
- **Lockdowns and their impact on mental health:** The implementation of lockdowns to slow the spread of the virus has had a significant impact on mental health, leading to increased levels of stress, anxiety, and depression. There has been debate over the effectiveness of lockdowns as a public health measure and the impact they have had on mental health and the economy. During the next pandemic, such decisions should be data driven modulated by public health experts.

These are just a few of the controversies and debates surrounding the COVID-19 pandemic. The pandemic has highlighted the need for effective and coordinated global action, as well as the importance of transparent and accurate information sharing.

4.1 Big-Tech Fights during COVID

During the COVID-19 pandemic, the role of big technology companies has come under increased scrutiny, with several controversies emerging related to their actions and policies. Some of the key fights between big tech companies and various stakeholders during the pandemic include:

Privacy concerns: There has been criticism of technology companies collecting and using large amounts of data related to the pandemic, including location data, health data, and personal information. Some privacy advocates have raised concerns about the potential misuse of this data and the lack of transparency and accountability around its collection and use.

Disinformation: The spread of misinformation and conspiracy theories related to the pandemic has led to several controversies, particularly on social media platforms. There has been criticism of the role of technology companies in amplifying false and dangerous information and the lack of action taken to remove such content from their platforms.

Antitrust issues: The COVID-19 pandemic has brought increased attention to the concentration of power and market share in the technology industry, leading to increased scrutiny of the practices of big technology companies. There have been allegations of anti-competitive behaviour, including the abuse of dominant market positions, which calls for greater regulation of the tech industry. These issues will be amplified by the use of artificial intelligence which operate behind the walls with transparency being knocked out of the ground.

Remote work and employee treatment: The shift to remote work as a result of the pandemic has also led to controversy, with criticism of the conditions and treatment of remote workers, particularly those in the gig economy. There have also been concerns about the impact of remote work on mental health and the need for better support and protection for remote workers.

Government collaboration: There have been controversies surrounding the collaboration of big tech companies with governments, particularly regarding the provision of technology and data to assist with tracking and controlling the spread of the virus. Some privacy advocates have raised concerns about the potential for such collaboration to be used for surveillance and other unethical purposes.

4.2 Vaccine Efficacy

A vaccine's efficacy is demonstrated in its ability to prevent the transmission of the virus from one person to another. If an exposed person does not contract the virus, they will, by definition, not develop symptoms or disease.

Prevention of Severe Disease: A vaccine's efficacy is also measured by its ability to prevent an exposed person from developing severe symptoms that may require hospitalization or lead to death. For each of the outcomes above, we also capture the differences by:

- Baseline vaccine effectiveness after second dose, waning immunity considering time since vaccination, and booster dose efficacy;
- Vaccine type: Pfizer & BioNTech (BNT162b2), Moderna (mRNA-1279), AstraZeneca (ChAdOx1), Janssen (Ad26.COV2.S), and other vaccines with available results;
- Variant of COVID-19: D614G (ancestral type), B.1.1.7 (Alpha), B.1.351 (Beta), P.1 (Gamma), B.1.617.2 (Delta), and B.1.1.529 (Omicron).

https://www.healthdata.org/covid/press-releases

JAMA study: Women are twice as likely as men to develop long COVID

https://www.healthdata.org/node/8584

Did the vaccines prevent transmission or prevented severe disease after infection?

COVID-19 vaccines probably were effective in preventing severe disease and saving lives, while their role in preventing transmission was secondary and less durable, especially with the emergence of immune-evasive variants.

4.3 The efficacy of Indian COVID-19 vaccines

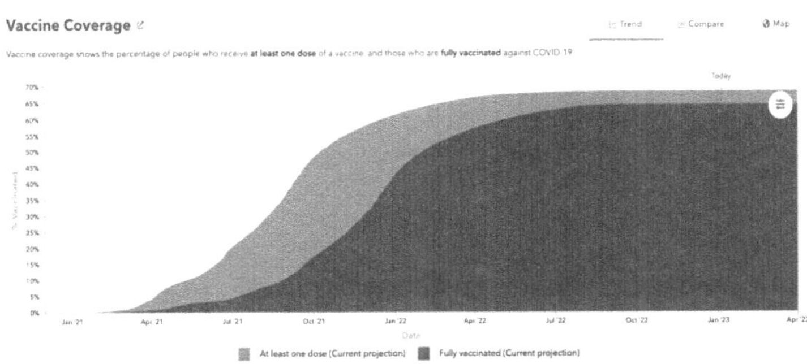

Figure 4.1 Dynamics of vaccine coverage

Covaxin (BBV152) and Covishield (ChAdOx1 nCoV-19), has been studied extensively: In clinical trials, Covaxin showed an efficacy of 77.8% in preventing symptomatic COVID-19. Real-world studies reported its efficacy against severe disease ranging between 69% and 78%, particularly against the Delta variant. Covaxin may be less effective in preventing infection but provides robust protection against severe illness.

4.3.1 Covishield:

Covishield demonstrated an efficacy of nearly 80% against severe disease in real-world scenarios. Its effectiveness varied between 54% and 95% depending on factors such as the timing of doses and regional variations. Like Covaxin, it has significantly reduced severe cases and hospitalizations.

All Indians received the vaccination through the COWIN app and all the RT-PCR tests were all also digitally registered. This was our best opportunity to understand the real-world efficacy of the vaccines used in India. Have we been up to the mark to analyze the data and generate meaningful information?

4.4 Healthy vaccine bias

> ⓘ Note
>
> The author in (44) revealed a dangerous truth about the vaccine booster effectiveness. The report indicates that the adjusted 90% lower mortality due to COVID-19 reported among the participants who received a booster cannot, with certainty, be attributed to boosting. "Healthy vaccine bias" in this population may have also led to overestimates of vaccine effectiveness in similar studies from Clalit Health Services. Inclusion of mortality not related to COVID-19 in all observational COVID-19 vaccine studies would provide an important context.

4.5 COVID and the geopolitics

The COVID-19 pandemic has significantly impacted elections in democracies and is likely to continue to do so in the future. Some of the ways in which COVID-19 has affected elections include:

- **Changes to voting methods**. The government has introduced several changes to voting methods to make it easier for people to vote during the pandemic. These include increased postal voting, extended proxy voting, and the introduction of voting by telephone.
- **Reduced voter turnout**. Some evidence suggests that voter turnout has decreased in elections held during the pandemic. This is likely due to a number of factors, including concerns about public health, logistical challenges, and the need for more awareness of the changes to voting methods.
- **Shifting political priorities**. The pandemic has also led to a shift in political priorities. Voters are now more likely to be concerned about issues such as the economy, healthcare, and public safety. This could have an impact on the outcome of future elections.

4.6 How is COVID-19 likely to affect future elections?

Since the public memory is short, we may assume that the traumatic days of the pandemic will be forgotten and the future elections will be unaffected by the dreadful days of COVID-19 infection. However, this may not be the case. The recent enquiries on mismanagement during the COVID-

19 days has changed the course of elections, even in countries like the UK. The COVID enquiries underway in the UK could have had a significant impact on the last general election. The enquiries were investigating the government's handling of the pandemic, and they could uncover evidence of mismanagement or negligence. The enquiries were also focusing on the issue of "Partygate", which refers to the allegations that government officials held parties during the COVID-19 lockdown. The findings damaged the reputation of the Conservative Party and made it more difficult for them to win the next election. The possibility of impacts of future political equations can not be ruled out even for superpowers like the US or China. The COVID-19 pandemic has exposed the vulnerabilities of superpowers and has led to a reassessment of their respective positions in the world.

The COVID-19 pandemic has highlighted the importance of biosecurity. If it is found that the virus originated from the Wuhan lab, it could lead to a renewed focus on this issue. Countries may be more likely to invest in biosecurity measures, and there could be increased cooperation between countries on this issue.

In the 2024 U.S. presidential election, there was a notable decrease in voter turnout in some areas, such as Chicago, which experienced its second-lowest voter turnout in the last 80 years. This decline may be attributed to the overwhelming number of choices and issues that voters faced, leading to decision fatigue and reduced participation. The pandemic has also influenced political outcomes by highlighting health care as a critical issue. The recent US elections has shown certain swings and the COVID-19 crisis might have played a role in the people's verdict in USA. In the 2024 U.S. elections, health care issues, including the handling of the pandemic and health care inequality, played a significant role in shaping voter preferences. The pandemic's impact on public health and the economy has been a focal point in political campaigns, with candidates addressing these concerns to appeal to voters. Some of the post electoral declarations by the new president-elect is a proof of this health-focus.

4.7 Covid Vaccine in Indian Election 2024

As expected, the vaccine controversy was also raised in the Indian parliamentary elections. The term Thrombosis with Thrombocytopenia Syndrome (TTS) is a rare yet serious condition linked to certain COVID-19 vaccines, notably adenovirus vector vaccines like AstraZeneca and Johnson & Johnson's Janssen vaccine and is trending in X-handles of certain political establishments. However, the point here is best explained by Google's Gemini. The chance of thrombocytopenia (low platelet count) with Covishield is very rare. Reports suggest an incidence of around 0.61 to 10 cases per million vaccine doses [Indian Express, Hindustan Times]. This translates to a very low probability. To give you an idea, the risk of a serious car accident is significantly higher. While the benefits of Covishield in preventing severe COVID-19 far outweigh the sporadic risk of thrombocytopenia, TTP is undoubtedly helping the swing of votes in favour or against a certain political establishment in India. On a lighter note, this is an excellent example of nonlinear dynamics and chaos, where an extremely low probability event can cause mass-scale change in public perception of the event. According to the X-handle *@harryminat*, when parliamentary questions were asked in the European Union regarding the cause of death following COVID-19 vaccines, 8368 of the 11,448 deaths were following the Pfizer Vaccine. On the other hand, had 80% of the 250 crore jabs by COVISHIELD followed a similar statstics of side effects half of them would have died of heart attack. The reelection of the previous NDA in 2024 suggested that challenges posed by the COVID-19 could not greatly affect the Indian electoral process. This also implied that Indian adaptations in logistics, campaign strategies, and voter engagement despite the post-pandemic hurdles, played a significant role. India's elections continue to reflect the vibrant democratic spirit of the country, with significant attention on economic issues and governmental responses to the pandemic.

4.8 The COVID-19 in future textbooks

COVID-19 will likely be looked upon in future textbooks of the history of medicine as a watershed moment. It was the first global-scale pandemic of the 21st century, profoundly impacting how we live and work. Textbooks will likely discuss the following aspects of COVID-19. Here are some 2024 books, (45,46), that would set the template of how the future texts would look like. Future textbooks may analyze the COVID-19 pandemic as a historical event, comparing it to past pandemics and discussing its place in history (like the Table 1.3 of our book). They might explore how different countries responded to the crisis and the lessons learned for future global health emergencies. The pandemic's impact on global politics and international relations could also be a significant area of study for future policy makers.

4.8.1 Positives

- The rapid spread of the virus and the challenges it posed to public health systems around the world gave rise to new ideas of tracking and intervening.
- The development of vaccines and treatments and the ethical debates surrounding them.
- The social and economic impact of the pandemic, including the rise of remote work and the economic disparities that were exacerbated by the crisis.
- COVID-19 will also be remembered as a time of great innovation in medicine. The development of vaccines and treatments in record time was a testament to the ingenuity of scientists and doctors around the world.
- The pandemic also highlighted the importance of public health measures, such as social distancing and mask-wearing. These measures were effective in slowing the spread of the virus, and they will likely be used in future pandemics.

4.8.2 Negatives

- COVID-19 may encourage some people to engage in the development of bioweapon(s) using DNA or RNA technology, a no less evil scenario than nuclear proliferation.
- The grey areas and loopholes in public health management are now wide open. It needs policymakers with a 360-degree vision to deal with disaster management of this magnitude.

- Social media can play the role of Frankenstein and contribute to the infodemic with disastrous effects

4.9 DTP vaccine and conspiracy theory

Conspiracy theories surrounding vaccines, including the DTP vaccine, have historically contributed to vaccine hesitancy and mistrust in public health institutions. These theories often claim that vaccines are harmful or part of a larger conspiracy, which can lead to skepticism about new vaccines, such as those for COVID-19. For instance, the belief that vaccines cause autism, despite being debunked by numerous studies, has persisted and influenced public perception of vaccine safety. DTP (Diphtheria-Tetanus-Pertussis) was associated with increased mortality among African children. The paper (47) concluded that DTP was associated with increased mortality among children; OPV (oral polio vaccine), however, minimized the effect of DTP. The referred study and cleaning of the original data was supported by a common grant from DANIDA and the Novo Nordisk Foundation (FU-11-551).

> ⓘ Note
>
> DANIDA report was criticized by Bill Gates (who funded the DTP vaccination program), calling it "deeply flawed".

However, having better nutritional status and being protected against three infections, 6–35-month-old DTP-vaccinated children tended to have higher mortality than DTP-unvaccinated children. This was re-confirmed by an additional report (48). There are always two sides of the coin.

Technology and AI should help us find more answers than raise further questions

4.10 Impact of conspiracy theories on the COVID-19 Narratives

The spread of conspiracy theories has led to a significant increase in vaccine hesitancy. Many people who believe in these theories are less likely to trust COVID-19 vaccines, viewing them with suspicion and fear. This hesitancy is not only a barrier to achieving herd immunity but also contributes to the spread of misinformation about the pandemic.

Public Health Challenges: The prevalence of conspiracy theories has made it challenging for public health officials to communicate effectively about the safety and efficacy of COVID-19 vaccines. This trend can lead to reduced vaccination rates, as seen in various regions where vaccine hesitancy is on the rise. Lastly what seems as conspiracy theory to some may appear as truth to some other groups and labelling the entire spectrum of conspiracy theorists as anti-science may be unfair and we cannot afford to be dogmatic

4.11 Vaccines as a Bioweapon

In an earlier section (Chapter 3), we mentioned how infections could be weaponized (the earliest example being the intentional propagation of smallpox among the native Indian population by the invaders). The role of invaders has now been replaced by big corporate and pharma houses and authoritarian governments. You can read about the criticism of HPV initiatives by Gates Foundation (https://economictimes.indiatimes.com/industry/healthcar

e/biotech/healthcare/controversial-vaccine-studies-why-is-bill-melinda-gates-foundation-under-fire-from-critics-in-india/articleshow/41280050.cms?from=mdr)

4.12 Claims and counterclaims on the use of COVID-19 vaccine as a bioweapon

Miles Guo not only alerted the FBI in 2017 about the planned CCP's bioweapon attack but also warned the public in 2019 that the emerging respiratory outbreak had human-to-human transmission and in January 2020 that it was caused by the CCP's bioweapon released by the military. He also predicted how the discovery process would unfold. Guo has also promoted the use of unproven treatments for COVID-19, such as artemisinin and ivermectin. These treatments have not been shown to be effective against COVID-19, and they can have serious side effects. Scientists and medical experts have widely criticized Guo's claims about COVID-19. They have warned that Guo's misinformation is dangerous and could lead to people avoiding effective treatments or taking unproven treatments that could harm them. In March 2023, Guo was arrested in the United States for fraud and money laundering charges. He is currently being held in jail without bail.

> ⓘ Note
>
> Miles is still locked in the US jail, with no bail allowed. Some believe that this persecution has been done by the CCP and its globalist co-conspirators.

Similarly, the Russian allegation in the United Nations that Ukrainian and American authorities collaborated to make a bioweapon laboratory targeting the African and Russian populations in Ukraine was junked by the UN experts. The only politician who has raised some serious concerns over this matter is RF Kennedy JR. According to him, the term 'misinformation' was coined to describe information that FaceBook and Twitter understood was true but that the WHO and other federal agencies wanted to be censored anyway for political reasons because it challenged official orthodoxies. RF Kennedy JR who has now been appointed as the Health Secretary of the USA has written a number of books on this subject which makes interesting reading

Table 4.1 COVID-19 origins and claims and debunking

Date	**Source**	**Claim**	**Debunked by**
Jan 2020	Washington Times	Virus was part of a Chinese biological weapons program based at the WIV	BBC, Washington Post
Feb 2020	U.S. Senator Tom Cotton	Virus may have been a Chinese bioweapon	Financial Times
Mar 2020	Financial Times	No evidence of genetic engineering, mutations	Dr Trevor Bedford

Date	Source	Claim	Debunked by
		consistent with natural evolution	
Mar2022	Russian Ministry of Defense	Ukrainian bioweapons lab owned by Hunter Biden	Junked by US and United Nations
March 2023	Google	Negative effects of vaccine and benefits of artemisinin and ivermectin	US authorities
July 2023	Twitter-travis_in_flint	151 percent increase in Myocarditis after the vaccine rollouts for US military	Case unsettled despite confirmation from Pentagon officials

The bio-weapon angle would thus remain as mysterious as the UFO. Certain problems are non-solvable, and this is one of them. Perhaps a future geopolitical realignment and declassification of documents may unfold some of the real stories behind this pandemic.

5.
How Covid Has Changed the Course of Genomic Research

The COVID-19 pandemic has accelerated the development and use of single-cell research in vaccine design. Single-cell analysis allows scientists to study the immune response at the level of individual cells, providing insights into how different vaccines work and how they can be improved.

5.1 Boost in single-cell research

Some important goals of single-cell research in vaccine design include:

- **Identifying new vaccine targets:** Single-cell analysis can be used to identify new antigens that could be used to develop vaccines. For example, a study published in 2021 used single-cell analysis to identify novel antigens from the SARS-CoV-2 virus that could be used to develop more effective vaccines.
- **Understanding the immune response to vaccines:** Single-cell analysis can be used to understand how different vaccines work and how they can be improved. For example, a study published in 2022 (49) used single-cell analysis to study the immune response to the COVID-19 vaccine from Pfizer-BioNTech. This research showed that the vaccine elicits a strong and diverse

immune response, including both humoral (antibody-mediated) and cellular (T-cell-mediated) immunity.

- **Personalizing vaccines:** Single-cell analysis can be used to identify biomarkers that are associated with the immune response to a particular vaccine (50). These biomarkers could then be used to identify individuals who are more likely to respond to the vaccine. Single-cell analysis can also be used to understand how the immune system responds to a particular vaccine. This information could be used to design vaccines that are more effective at stimulating the immune system. Single-cell analysis can also be used to tailor vaccines to the individual patient's immune system. This could involve using different vaccine components or delivery methods for patients.

5.2 Pfizer-BioNTech initiatives

The Pfizer-BioNTech COVID-19 vaccine was one of the first vaccines to be developed using single-cell analysis. This vaccine was designed to target a specific antigen of the SARS-CoV-2 virus, which was identified using single-cell analysis. The vaccine has been shown to be highly effective at preventing COVID-19 and is credited with helping to save millions of lives.

5.3 Initiatives from DARPA

The Defense Advanced Research Projects Agency (DARPA) has funded several initiatives to develop new methods for single-cell research. These initiatives include:

- **The Cell-Centric Immune Defenses (CCID) program:** This program is focused on developing new methods for studying the immune system at the single-cell level. The goal is to develop new insights into how the immune system responds to infection and disease.
- **The Single Cell Analysis for Biomedical Applications (SCABa) program:** This program is focused on developing new technologies and methods for analyzing single-cell data. The goal of this program is to make single-cell analysis more accessible and to enable new discoveries in biomedical research.
- **The Single Cell Abundance and Function (SCAF) program:** This program is focused on developing new methods for measuring the abundance and function of single cells in complex tissues. This program aims to develop new tools for studying the heterogeneity of tissues and improve our understanding of how tissues function.

These initiatives are helping to accelerate the development of single-cell research and to make this powerful technology more accessible to scientists. This is likely to significantly impact the future of vaccine development and other areas of biomedical research.

5.4 Development of mRNA anti-cancer vaccine by Russia

On the website of the National Medical Research Centre of the Russian Ministry of Health, there is a one-paragraph description of the work of the Russian researchers with regards to the development of the anti-cancer mRNA vaccine. It says that the "personalized mRNA vaccines" will be based on the genetic analysis of each person's tumor on a "unique software platform" to identify the mutations called neoantigens.

(https://indianexpress.com/article/explained/explained-health/russia-vaccine-cancer-9744034/)

6.
How Climate Patterns Were Affected by COVID-19 Related Measures

A critical review (51) discussed the climatic effect of the COVID-19 Pandemic. Olusula et al (52) have discussed the impact of the COVID-19 pandemic on nitrogen dioxide levels in Nigeria. The greenhouse gas level changes were extensively discussed by (53). Primary emissions of criteria pollutants and greenhouse gases during COVID-19 pandemic disruptions were discussed by (54). A study by (55) revealed that NO2, a major pollutant emitted by vehicles, and SO2, emitted by power plants, underwent significant changes during the peak of the pandemic. The study used Ozone Monitoring Instrument (OMI) data and Atmospheric Infrared Sounder (AIRS) satellites.

The study found that reductions in air pollution were most pronounced in urban areas and during the daytime. For example, during the lockdown period, NO2 levels decreased by up to 50% in New Delhi, India. In Beijing, China, SO2 levels decreased by up to 30%.

The study's findings suggest that COVID-19 lockdowns had a significant impact on air pollution levels. This is important because air pollution is a major contributor to climate change and respiratory diseases.

The COVID-19 pandemic has had a significant impact on climate patterns. The measures taken to mitigate the spread of the virus, such as lockdowns and travel restrictions, have led to a decrease in greenhouse gas emissions and air pollution. This has resulted in a temporary improvement in air quality and a decrease in the rate of climate change. For example, a study by the University of California, Berkeley found that global emissions of nitrogen dioxide, a pollutant that contributes to smog and acid rain, fell by 40% in the first few months of the pandemic. The study also found that air quality in many cities improved significantly during this time.

However, it is essential to note that the positive effects of the COVID-19 measures on climate patterns are likely to be temporary. As the world economy recovers and people start to travel and move around more, emissions are likely to start rising again. *Revenge travel* has actually made matters worse.

In addition, the pandemic has also had some adverse effects on climate patterns. For example, the decrease in air traffic has led to a decrease in contrails, which are condensation trails that form behind jet planes. Contrails can reflect sunlight and help to cool the Earth's atmosphere. The decrease in contrails has led to a slight increase in global temperatures.

Overall, the impact of the COVID-19 pandemic on climate patterns is complex and multifaceted. There have been both positive and negative effects, and it is too early to say what the long-term consequences will be.

Here are some of the specific ways in which climate patterns have been affected by COVID-19-related measures:

1. **Air quality has improved**. The decrease in air traffic and other human activities has decreased air pollution, improving air quality in many cities.
2. **The rate of climate change has slowed**. The decrease in greenhouse gas emissions has slowed the rate of climate change. However, it is essential to note that this is a temporary effect, and emissions will likely start rising again as the world economy recovers.
3. **The frequency and intensity of extreme weather events have increased**. Some studies have shown that the frequency and intensity of extreme weather events, such as heatwaves, droughts, and floods, have increased during the COVID-19 pandemic. However, it is unclear whether this is due to the pandemic or other factors, such as climate change.

The long-term effects of the COVID-19 pandemic on climate patterns are still uncertain and require further research.

6.1 Air Quality Standards (NAAQS)

The following table compares the National Ambient Air Quality Standards (NAAQS) with current prevailing levels for several pollutants:

Table 5.1 Recommended versus pollutant level during the pandemic

Pollutant	NAAQS Recommendation	Levels during the pandemic
Carbon monoxide (CO)	9 ppm annual average	1.7 ppm
Lead (Pb)	0.15 μg/m³ annual average	0.003 μg/m³
Nitrogen dioxide (NO2)	0.053 ppm annual average	0.039 ppm
Ozone (O3)	0.075 ppm annual average	0.067 ppm
Particulate matter (PM10)	150 μg/m³ 24-hour average	39 μg/m³
Particulate matter (PM2.5)	12.0 μg/m³ annual average	10 μg/m³

The level of CO was 1.7 ppm, which was below the NAAQS of 9 ppm. This is true for most other pollutants. This means that air quality in many parts of the world met the EPA's CO standards. However, it is essential to note that the NAAQS is designed to be protective, and so even though the level of CO was below the NAAQS, it is still possible that there could be some harm at this level.

6.2 CO dynamics during COVID

The following graph shows the CO levels in different COVID-19 states:

```
# Load the R library 'ggplot2'
library(ggplot2)

# Create a data frame with the CO level and year
data <- data.frame(year = c(2019, 2020, 2021, 2022, 2023),
                   co_level = c(1.7, 1.3, 1.5, 1.6, 1.7))

# Create a line plot of the CO level by year
plt<- ggplot(data, aes(x = year, y = co_level)) +
  geom_point(alpha = 0.5) +
  geom_line(linetype = "dashed") +
  labs(title = "CO Level by Year",
       x = "Year",
       y = "CO Level (ppm)") +
  geom_abline(intercept = 1.3, slope = 0, linetype = "dashed", color
= "red") +
  geom_abline(intercept = 1.5, slope = 0, linetype = "dashed", color
= "red") +
  geom_abline(intercept = 1.6, slope = 0, linetype = "dashed", color
= "red")
ggsave("./images/CO_Level_by_Year.png", plot = plt, width = 6, h
eight = 4, dpi = 300)
```

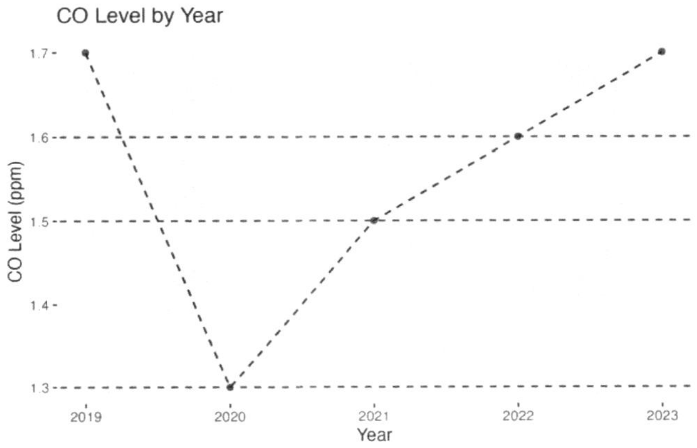

Figure 6.1 CO-level by year

The graph shows that CO levels decreased significantly during the COVID-19 pandemic. The levels have since rebounded somewhat but are still below pre-pandemic levels.

The findings of this study suggest that COVID-19 lockdowns can have a significant impact on air pollution levels. This is important because air pollution is a major contributor to climate change and respiratory diseases.

The study also highlights the importance of monitoring air pollution levels during times of crisis. This will help us to understand the impact of different interventions on air quality and to develop strategies to mitigate the effects of air pollution.

6.3 A comprehensive dynamic of different pollutants before and after COVID

```
library(ggplot2)

# Create a data frame with the pollutant levels and year
data <- data.frame(
  year = c(2019, 2020, 2021, 2022, 2023),
  co_level = c(1.7, 1.3, 1.5, 1.6, 1.7),
  pb_level = c(0.003, 0.002, 0.002, 0.003, 0.004),
  no2_level = c(0.039, 0.035, 0.032, 0.036, 0.038),
  so2_level = c(0.067, 0.062, 0.058, 0.064, 0.066),
  pm10_level = c(39, 36, 33, 37, 38)
)

# Calculate the fractional change of each pollutant
data$co_frac_change <- (data$co_level - data$co_level[1]) / data
$co_level[1]
data$pb_frac_change <- (data$pb_level - data$pb_level[1]) / data
$pb_level[1]
```

```
data$no2_frac_change <- (data$no2_level - data$no2_level[1]) /
data$no2_level[1]
data$so2_frac_change <- (data$so2_level - data$so2_level[1]) / d
ata$so2_level[1]
data$pm10_frac_change <- (data$pm10_level - data$pm10_level[
1]) / data$pm10_level[1]

# Reshape the data into a long format using pivot_longer
data_long <-
 tidyr::pivot_longer(
  data, cols =
   c(co_frac_change, pb_frac_change, no2_frac_change, so2_frac
_change, pm10_frac_change),
  names_to = "pollutant",
  values_to = "frac_change"
)

# Plot the fractional change of each pollutant
plt<- ggplot(data_long, aes(x = year, y = frac_change, color = po
llutant)) +
  geom_line(size = 1.5) +
  labs(title = "Fractional Change of Air Pollutant Levels",
      x = "Year",
      y = "Fractional Change") +
  theme_bw() +
  theme(legend.position = "bottom")
```

```
Warning: Using `size` aesthetic for lines was deprecated in ggplot
2 3.4.0.
i Please use `linewidth` instead.
```

```
ggsave("./images/many_pollutants.png", plot = plt, width = 6, h
eight = 4, dpi = 300)
```

6.4 Interpretation of the V-shaped pollutant curve

The onset of COVID had the fastest impact on the two pollutants, CO and Pb (this instant behaviour may be traced back to the less use of automobiles). The Pb strikingly was not restored in the post-COVID period, but other pollutants did. The NO2 and the PM10 responded with a time delay, indicating the involvement of some atmospheric processes.

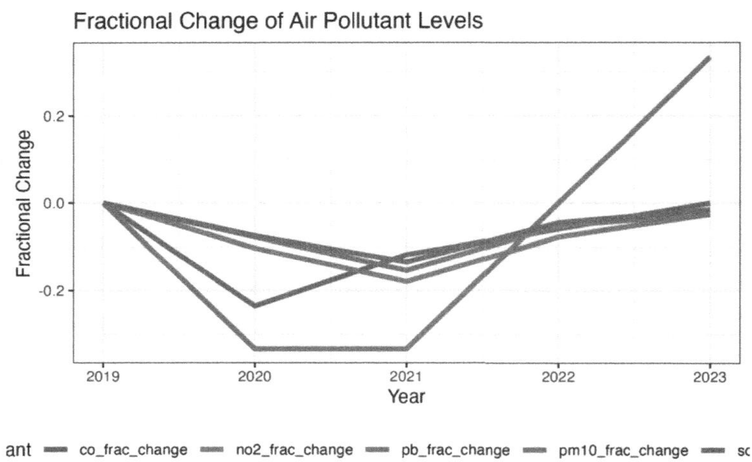

Figure 6.2 Various pollutants by Year

Appendix I

We have tried to discuss some elements of the COVID-19 pandemic which will help us develop the cheat sheet for management of the next crisis in a better way.

AI.1 Mental Health and COVID-19:

The psychological impact of the pandemic on individuals and communities, the rise in mental health issues, and the importance of mental health support during challenging times has impacted humanity in a major way which perhaps we couldn't have predicted earlier [1]Despite various debates on the issue, it is universally accepted that the COVID-19 pandemic has had profound effects on mental health globally, exacerbating existing issues and creating new challenges. Several factors contributed to the mental health

---

[1] The pandemic has led to an increase in anxiety and depression. Studies have shown that up to 40% of people have experienced symptoms of anxiety or depression during the pandemic. The pandemic has also led to an increase in suicide rates. In the United States, suicide rates increased by 15% in 2020. The pandemic has had a disproportionate impact on certain groups of people, such as young people, women, and people of colour. These groups are more likely to experience anxiety, depression, and suicidal thoughts. The pandemic has also disrupted access to mental health care. Many people have lost their jobs or had their hours reduced, making it difficult to afford mental health care. In addition, many mental health providers have had to reduce their services or close their practices altogether.

crisis, including social isolation, financial instability, fear of infection, and grief from loss. Vulnerable groups such as healthcare workers, individuals with pre-existing mental health conditions, and economically disadvantaged populations were disproportionately affected. Some of the critical issues associated are:

- **Increased Anxiety and Depression**: The uncertainty surrounding the pandemic led to a surge in anxiety disorders and depression. Studies show that these conditions significantly increased during lockdowns, with many reporting feelings of hopelessness and despair.
- **Rise in Post-Traumatic Stress Disorder (PTSD):** A vast majority of patients infected with the Coronavirus recovered, but some of them—in the range of 6.2% to 45% —go on to develop long COVID. Of them, approximately 30% develop frank PTSD) or PTSD symptoms, but figures of approximately 50% have also been reported. Affected persons included Healthcare workers, COVID-19 survivors, and those grieving the loss of loved ones who experienced symptoms of PTSD due to prolonged exposure to trauma.
- **Social Isolation**: Quarantine measures and social distancing disrupted regular social interactions, leading to loneliness and a decline in overall emotional well-being.
- **Substance Abuse**: Many individuals turned to alcohol and drugs as coping mechanisms, leading to increased substance abuse cases globally.

- **Impact on Children and Adolescents**: The closure of schools and disruption of routines led to increased anxiety, behavioral issues, and academic challenges among children and teenagers.

AI.2 Social and Economic Impacts:

Social and economic consequences of the pandemic include unemployment, poverty, inequality, and the challenges faced by different sectors. The COVID-19 pandemic has had a profound impact on societies and economies worldwide.

Social Consequences

- Disruption of education: School closures and remote learning have disrupted the education of millions of children and young people, with potential long-term consequences for their academic and social development.
- Exacerbation of inequalities: The pandemic has disproportionately affected marginalized and vulnerable groups, such as low-income individuals, racial and ethnic minorities, and people with disabilities.
- Global recession: The pandemic triggered a global recession, leading to job losses, business closures, and decreased economic activity.
- Increased unemployment: Many industries, including tourism, hospitality, and retail, experienced significant job losses due to lockdowns and reduced consumer spending.

- Supply chain disruptions: The pandemic disrupted global supply chains, leading to shortages of essential goods and increased prices.
- Sector-Specific Challenges Healthcare: Healthcare systems were overwhelmed, leading to delays in treatment for non-COVID-19 conditions and increased healthcare worker burnout.
- Education: The shift to remote learning has highlighted digital divides and inequities in education access.
- Tourism and hospitality: The tourism and hospitality industries were among the most brutal hit, with widespread job losses and business closures.
- Retail: The pandemic accelerated the shift to online shopping, leading to challenges for traditional brick-and-mortar retailers.
- Manufacturing: Supply chain disruptions and decreased demand have impacted the manufacturing sector.
- Governments and international organizations have implemented various measures to mitigate the social and economic impacts of the pandemic, including fiscal stimulus packages, job support programs, and social safety nets.

Economic consequences:

- The pandemic has had a significant impact on the global economy, leading to recessions and job losses in many countries. The tourism industry has been particularly hard hit, as people have been reluctant to travel during the pandemic. Many businesses have also been forced to close or downsize, leading to job losses and increased poverty. The pandemic has also had a negative impact on global trade, as countries have imposed travel restrictions and closed borders. Social consequences: The pandemic has led to an increase in isolation and loneliness, as people have been forced to stay home and avoid contact with others. This has hurt mental health, as people have struggled to cope with the stress of the pandemic. The pandemic has also led to an increase in domestic violence, as people have been spending more time at home with their partners. The pandemic has also had a negative impact on education, as schools have been closed and children have been forced to learn from home.

AI.3 Vaccination Strategies:

Different vaccination strategies adopted by countries, challenges in vaccine distribution, vaccine hesitancy, and the role of vaccination in controlling the pandemic. [3]. Countries

---

[3] The type of vaccine: Different types of vaccines have different safety profiles. For example, live attenuated vaccines (which contain a weakened form of the virus) are more likely to cause side effects than inactivated vaccines (which do not contain any live virus). The long-term effects of mRNA vaccines are not yet known, as these vaccines have only been in use for a relatively short period of time. So, a detailed study of vaccinated individuals is needed. The vaccine recipient's age: The vaccine's safety may vary depending on the age of the vaccine recipient. For example, some vaccines are not

worldwide have adopted diverse strategies to combat the COVID-19 pandemic through vaccination.

- United States: Large-scale vaccination centers, pharmacies, and community clinics were established.
- United Kingdom: A rapid rollout involving GP surgeries, mass vaccination centers, and mobile units.
- India: A massive vaccination drive, especially in rural areas, utilizing a vast network of healthcare providers.
- Israel: Prioritized vaccination of older adults and healthcare workers.
- Singapore: A phased approach, starting with healthcare workers and vulnerable populations.
- Australia: A cautious and phased approach, initially focusing on frontline workers and high-risk groups.
- China: Leveraged its strong public health infrastructure and digital technology for efficient vaccination campaigns.
- South Korea: Implemented a robust contact tracing system and used technology to monitor vaccination progress.

---

recommended for pregnant women or young children. The underlying health conditions of the vaccine recipient: People with underlying health conditions may be at an increased risk of side effects from some vaccines.

AI.4 Long COVID:

We omitted the long-term effects of COVID-19 on individuals, known as "long COVID," and the challenges in managing and understanding this phenomenon. [4] Long COVID-19, or post-COVID-19 condition, is a complex set of symptoms that can persist for months or even years after an initial COVID-19 infection. These symptoms can vary widely from person to person but may include fatigue, shortness of breath, brain fog, headaches, chest pain, anxiety, depression, and more. While the exact causes of Long COVID are still being researched, it is believed to be linked to the virus's impact on various organs and systems, including the lungs, heart, brain, and immune system.

---

[4] 14% of COVID-19 patients have elevated heart rates for months after infection. Long COVID is a wide range of new, returning, or ongoing health problems that people experience after being infected with the virus that causes COVID-19. Most people with COVID-19 get better within a few days to a few weeks after infection, so at least four weeks after infection, when Long COVID could first be identified. Anyone who is infected can experience Long COVID. Most people with Long COVID experienced symptoms days after first learning they had COVID-19, but some people who later experienced Long COVID did not know when they got infected. The silver lining is that COVID-19 infection after vaccination is less likely to report Long COVID than unvaccinated people.

AI.5 Ethical Dilemmas:

The COVID-19 pandemic presented numerous ethical dilemmas, particularly in the areas of resource allocation, public health measures, and individual rights. Here are some of the critical ethical challenges:

- Resource Allocation and prioritization of patients: With limited healthcare resources, difficult decisions had to be made about who would receive critical care, such as ventilators and ICU beds. This raised questions about fairness, equity, and potential bias.
- Age-based rationing: Some proposals suggested prioritizing younger, healthier individuals for scarce resources, leading to ethical debates about age discrimination and the value of human life.
- Disability-based rationing: Concerns arose about potential discrimination against individuals with disabilities, who might be seen as less deserving of care.

Public Health Measures:

- Balancing individual rights and public health: Implementing measures like lockdowns, quarantines, and mask mandates raised concerns about restrictions on personal freedoms and economic impact.
- Mandatory vaccination: Debates arose about whether governments should mandate vaccination to balance individual autonomy with the collective good.

- Surveillance and data privacy: Increased surveillance and data collection for contact tracing raised concerns about privacy rights and the potential for misuse of personal information.
- Informed consent: In the rush to develop and administer vaccines, ensuring fully informed consent for clinical trials and vaccinations became challenging.

Mental health impact: The pandemic's psychological toll led to increased mental health issues, raising questions about access to care and the ethical implications of treatment.

- Discrimination and stigma: Fear and misinformation led to discrimination against individuals with COVID-19 or those perceived as high-risk, impacting their social and economic well-being.

Addressing these ethical dilemmas required careful consideration of various factors, including:

- Equity: Ensuring fair distribution of resources and opportunities, particularly for marginalized groups.
- Transparency: Open and honest communication with the public about decision-making processes and the rationale behind policies.
- Accountability: Holding policymakers and healthcare providers accountable for their decisions and actions.

Among other ethical dilemmas raised during the pandemic, we must include some global-south-related issues, such as allocating resources and prioritizing vulnerable populations for vaccination. Balancing public health measures with individual rights perhaps demands more attention. [5]

AI.6 Mutations and Variants:

We did not provide a more detailed explanation of COVID-19 mutations and variants, their potential implications on transmission, severity, and vaccine efficacy, and how they have influenced public health strategies

---

[5] Support research on ethical issues: There is a need for more research on the ethical issues raised by the pandemic. This research will help us to understand these issues better and to develop more ethical ways to respond to future pandemics.

[6]Alpha: The Alpha variant was first identified in the United Kingdom in September 2020. It is thought to be more transmissible than the original strain of COVID-19, and it has been associated with an increased risk of hospitalization and death.https://www.news-medical.net/news/20211130/UK-study-finds-COVID-19-from-Delta-and-Alpha-infections-are-clinically-similar.aspx. Beta: The Beta variant was first identified in South Africa in December 2020. It is thought to be more transmissible than the original strain of COVID-19, and it has been associated with an increased risk of hospitalization.https://www.bbc.com/news/health-55534727.Gamma: The Gamma variant was first identified in Brazil in January 2021. It is thought to be more transmissible than the original strain of COVID-19, and it has been associated with an increased risk of hospitalization and death.https://www.mdpi.com/2076-393X/9/11/1305.Delta: The Delta variant was first identified in India in October 2020. It is the most transmissible variant of COVID-19 that has been identified so far, and it has been associated with an increased risk of hospitalization and death.https://www.emro.who.int/health-topics/corona-

AI.7 Long-Term Policy Recommendations:

If there is at all a long-term policy, that has to be evidence-based. This is a must for handling future pandemics. [7].

---

virus/delta-variant-social-media-cards.html.Omicron: The Omicron variant was first identified in South Africa in November 2021. It is the most mutated variant of COVID-19 that has been identified so far, and it is thought to be more transmissible than the Delta variant. However, whether Omicron is more severe than the Delta variant is unclear.https://www.pacehospital.com/omicron-variant-of-covid-19. It should be noted that information about variants from China is less known as the information sharing was minimal.

[7] Investment in research and development: Governments should invest in research and development to develop new vaccines, treatments, and diagnostics for COVID-19. This will help us to understand the virus better and to develop more effective ways to prevent, treat, and manage the disease. Strengthen global health systems: Governments should strengthen global health systems to better prepare for future pandemics. This includes investing in public health infrastructure, such as hospitals and clinics, and developing more robust surveillance systems to detect and respond to new outbreaks. Promote equity: Governments should promote equity in access to COVID-19 vaccines, treatments, and diagnostics. This means ensuring that everyone, regardless of their income or social status, has access to the tools they need to protect themselves and their families. Build public trust: Governments should build public trust in public health measures. This means being transparent about the risks of COVID-19 and the benefits of public health measures and ensuring that these measures are fair and equitable. Also, see sections 3.12-3.17 of the book for more detail. Prepare for the future: Governments should prepare for the future by developing contingency plans for future pandemics. This includes planning for

Table AI.1 Past Epidemic Experiences

Disease	Year(s)	Notes
H1N1 Influenza	2009	Declared as a PHEIC by WHO.
Ebola Virus Disease (EVD)	2014-2016, 2018-2020	Major outbreaks in West Africa and later in the Democratic Republic of Congo.
Zika Virus Disease (ZVD)	2016	Associated with birth defects like microcephaly.
Poliomyelitis	2014	Continued global efforts for eradication.
COVID-19	2020	Complex pandemic with recurring waves, mutations, and high public health impact.
Monkeypox	2022	Spread to non-endemic regions.
Severe Acute Respiratory Syndrome (SARS)	Early 2000s	Emerged in China; caused by a novel coronavirus.
Avian Influenza (Bird Flu)	Ongoing	Zoonotic disease with sporadic outbreaks.
Middle East Respiratory	2012 onwards	First identified in Saudi Arabia; linked to camels.

---

the distribution of vaccines, treatments, and diagnostics and the economic and social impacts of a pandemic.

Disease	Year(s)	Notes
Syndrome (MERS-CoV)		
Nipah Virus Outbreak	-	Sporadic outbreaks in South and Southeast Asia.

Key Initiative:

The **One Health (OH) Mission** by the Government of India aims to:

- Integrate human, animal, and environmental health sectors.

- Create a surveillance and outbreak response system.

- Focus on research to mitigate emerging zoonotic threats.

Appendix II

The recent announcement of Johns Hopkins University is that from March 2023.

Table AII.1 Data extracted from https://coronavirus.jhu.edu

Country	Confirmed Cases	Deaths	% Population with at least one vaccine dose
India	4,46,90,738	5,30,779	74.45%
USA	10,38,02,702	11,23,836	81.82%
China	49,03,524	1,01,056	92.81%
UK	2,46,58,705	2,20,721	79.27%

AII.1 Comment on PDI (Pandemic Data Initiative)

As associate vice provost for Public Sector Innovation at Johns Hopkins University (JHU), Beth Blauer oversees initiatives that help governments deploy data to maximize the delivery of public services. Blauer says she wants the Pandemic Data Initiative (PDI) to spur discussions about building a modern data collection infrastructure that would empower local, state, and federal agencies to execute a coordinated response for the next major public health crisis. As JHU announced the stoppage of data collection since March 2023, we may conclude the following: - No significant COVID cases since March 2023 - The JHU data collection program is no more sustainable

AII.2 Age structure of the COVID-19 death

According to the Centers for Disease Control and Prevention (CDC), the risk of death from COVID-19 for people aged 85 and older is 1 in 10. For people aged 65 to 74, the risk of death is 1 in 50. For people aged 55 to 64, the risk of death is 1 in 100. In contrast, the risk of death from COVID-19 for people under the age of 55 is much lower. For people aged 18 to 29, the risk of death is 1 in 10,000. For people aged 30 to 44, the risk of death is 1 in 5,000.

AII.3 Data Structure without clustering

However, let us look into an actual data set:

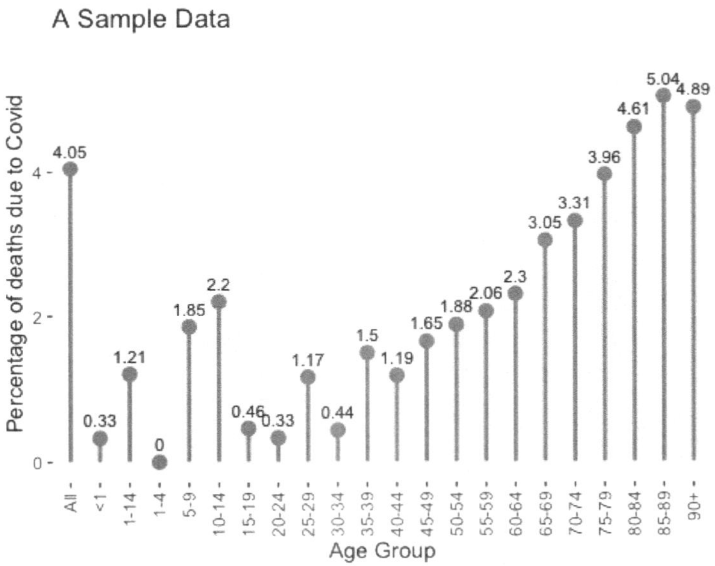

Figure AII.1 Age group dependence on percentage of death

AII.4 The need for a global data hunting

A global covid database is needed to understand the finer features of the pandemic. We need to understand the global trend and mutant specificity, if any, in case we have to arrive at a comprehensive COVID model. The other databases include Pandemic data initiative, our world data & Covid 19 data hub platform. [8,9,10]

Appendix III

AIII.1 Impact of COVID-19 on the epidemiology of malaria and dengue

Being a practising physician, one author (PC) witnessed that during the COVID peak, there were fewer occurrences of other infections, suggesting a cross-talk between different infections, such as COVID, Malaria and Dengue. His back-of-the-envelope estimation suggested that the number of malaria and dengue cases fell down since the start of the COVID-19 pandemic, and the non-covid outbreaks were restored to their default values once the COVID-19 infection subsided [11,12]

`geom_smooth()` using formula = 'y ~ x'

---

[11] The Impact of COVID-19 on Malaria: A Systematic Review: https://www.ncbi.nlm.nih.gov/pmc/articles/PMC8423804/. Dengue and COVID-19: A Syndemic in the Time of Global Pandemic: https://www.ncbi.nlm.nih.gov/pmc/articles/PMC8443888/.

[12] COVID-19 and the Risk of Coinfection with Other Mosquito-Borne Diseases: https://www.ncbi.nlm.nih.gov/pmc/articles/PMC8465774/

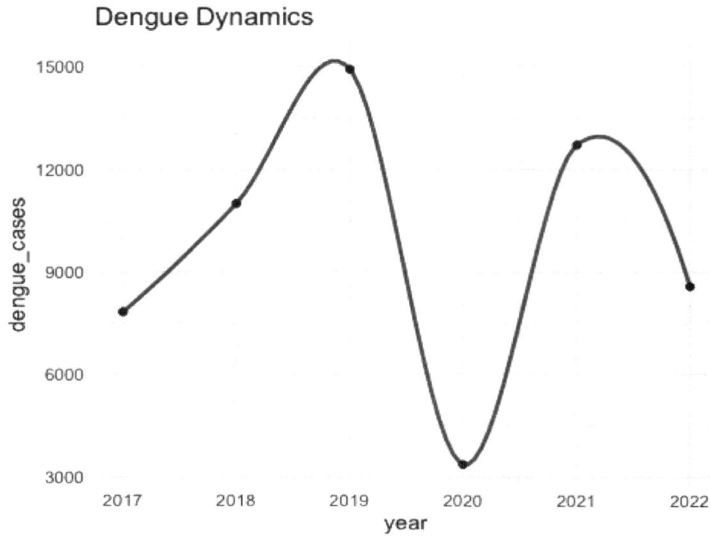

Figure AIII.1 Dengue dynamics

The gut observation by one of the authors matches with data from the state of Maharashtra, India. The outbreak of dengue was at 180 degrees phase-synced with COVID-19.

Appendix IV

When we started writing the book, the COVID wave started, but as we approached the book's completion, we saw someone getting a Nobel prize for the nucleoside base modifications that enabled the development of effective mRNA vaccines against COVID-19. Karikó and Weissman's work was essential to developing the mRNA vaccines that have been used to vaccinate billions of people worldwide against COVID-19. However, like many things in COVID, just after the declaration of the Nobel prize winner's name, a tweet appeared from Robert Malone:

> ⚠ Warning
>
> "Kariko and Weissman get the Nobel, not for inventing mRNA vaccines (because I did that) but for adding the pseudouridine that allowed unlimited spike toxins to be manufactured in what could have been a safe and effective vaccine platform if safely developed. Good to know." Robert Malone

Dr. Robert Malone is the inventor of mRNA vaccines. This collaborative effort began in the late 1980s when he introduced mRNA to human, rodent, frog, and fruit fly cells via liposomal nanoparticles. He and researchers from the University of Wisconsin, Madison, and Vical Incorporated injected naked RNA and DNA vectors into the skeletal muscle of mice and observed gene expression. Malone has argued that he was unfairly excluded from the Nobel Prize because of his involvement in the anti-vaccine movement.

Others have argued that Karikó and Weissman's work was essential to the development of mRNA vaccines, even though Malone made important contributions to the field. Karikó and Weissman's work on nucleoside base modifications was essential to making mRNA vaccines safe and effective.

The Nobel Prize Committee has defended its decision to award the prize to Karikó and Weissman, stating that their work was "crucial for developing effective mRNA vaccines against COVID-19". The committee also stated that it considered the contributions of all researchers who made significant contributions to the development of mRNA vaccines but that Karikó and Weissman's work was the most important. Whether this will be regarded as a geopolitically charged decision in the history of Nobel Prizes remains to be seen in the future.

AIV.1 The person (Malone) who pioneered the research on mRNA vaccine became an anti-vaxxer- why?

Pfizer mRNA vaccine is contaminated with plasmid DNA- 200 Billion Pieces of DNA in Each Dose. [https://twitter.com/i/status/1706859555194384633]. USC Professor Dr Philip Buckhaults warns of the severe side effects because of such plasmid leakage. The DNA can integrate into the genomic DNA of cells and poses a genuine theoretical future risk of cancer.

AIV.2 What is unique about mRNA vaccine as compared to traditional vaccines

Vaccination helps the body develop an immune response to a specific pathogen. This gives the body a head start in fighting off the disease if exposed to the pathogen later. Vaccines made from killed or weakened viruses have been around for a long time. Examples include the polio, measles, and yellow fever vaccines. Max Theiler (56) won the Nobel Prize in Physiology or Medicine in 1951 for developing the yellow fever vaccine.

In recent years, scientists have developed vaccines made from individual viral components instead of whole viruses. Parts of the viral genetic code, usually the parts that code for proteins on the virus's surface, are used to make proteins that trigger the production of virus-blocking antibodies using recombinant DNA technology. The hepatitis B and human papillomavirus vaccines are two examples. Another method is to transfer parts of the viral genetic code to a harmless carrier virus, called a "vector." This is done in Ebola vaccines (57). When vector vaccines are injected, the chosen viral protein is produced in our cells, which triggers an immune response against the target virus.

However, vaccine research underwent a tremendous change with the advent of the mRNA vaccine. Karikó and Weissman noticed that dendritic cells recognize in vitro transcribed mRNA as a foreign substance. Dendritic cells (DCs) are specialized antigen-presenting cells (APCs) crucial in initiating and orchestrating the immune response. They can recognize and capture a wide range of antigens, including in vitro transcribed mRNA (IVT mRNA). Such recognition leads to their activation and the release of inflammatory signaling molecules.

> ⓘ Note
>
> They wondered why the in vitro transcribed mRNA was recognized as foreign while mRNA from mammalian cells did not give rise to the same reaction. Karikó and Weissman realized that some critical properties must distinguish the different types of mRNA.

RNA from mammalian cells are frequently chemically modified, while in vitro transcribed mRNA is not. They wondered if the absence of altered bases in the in vitro transcribed RNA could explain the unwanted inflammatory reaction. To investigate this, they produced different variants of mRNA, each with unique chemical alterations in their bases, which they delivered to dendritic cells. The results were striking: The inflammatory response was almost abolished when base modifications were included in the mRNA. This was a paradigm change in our understanding of how cells recognize and respond to different forms of mRNA. Karikó and Weissman immediately understood that their discovery had profound significance for using mRNA as therapy. They started modifying the mRNA with pseudouridine. This explains why the claim by Dr. Robert Malone is not entirely true, as in his research, he missed this critical perspective of mRNA modification (58).

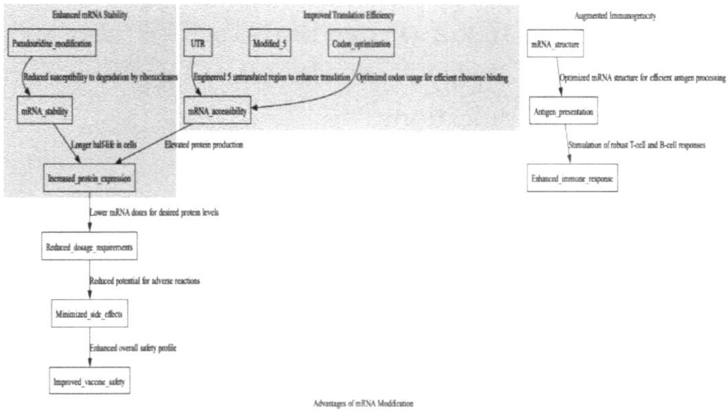

Figure AIV.1 Flow Chart Describing the advantages of mRNA modification

AIV.3 Risks of mRNA vaccine

Myocarditis: This is an inflammation of the heart muscle. It is a rare side effect of modified mRNA vaccines and is more common in young men. Post-mRNA vaccination myocarditis is seen predominantly in young males within a few days after their second vaccination dose. The pathophysiology of myocarditis is not well known (59). Pericarditis: This is an inflammation of the lining around the heart. It is also a rare side effect of modified mRNA vaccines and is more common in young men.

AIV.4 Differential Modifications in the mRNA vaccines

mRNA-1273: mRNA-1273 ((Moderna)) is capped with a 5' cap and a 3' poly-A tail. It also contains pseudouridine modifications, which help to stabilize the mRNA and make it less susceptible to degradation by ribonucleases. BNT162b2: BNT162b2 (Pfizer-BioNTech) is also capped with a 5' cap and a 3' poly-A tail. However, it does not contain pseudouridine modifications.

AIV.5 Legal issues

Even as recently as Nov 2023, there are emerging legal issues for the use of mRNA-modified vaccines, according to Attorney General Ken Paxton.

"Today, I have filed suit against Pfizer and Tris Pharma for defrauding Texas Medicaid and providing adulterating pharmaceuticals to children.

I am horrified by the dishonesty we uncovered in this investigation. Pfizer and Tris intentionally concealed and failed to disclose the issues with Quillivant receiving taxpayer-funded benefits through Texas Medicaid, defrauding the state and endangering children. Our Civil Medicaid Fraud Division has done an outstanding job holding these pharmaceutical companies accountable."

Appendix V

The Evolution of COVID-19 Management During the Pandemic

The COVID-19 pandemic presented unprecedented challenges to the global medical community. Over the course of the pandemic, the management of COVID-19 patients evolved significantly, driven by the rapid accumulation of scientific knowledge, the development of novel therapeutic strategies, and the experience gained from treating millions of patients worldwide.

AV.1 Early Phase: Uncertainty and Experimentation

1.1 Initial Management Strategies

- At the onset of the pandemic, the understanding of SARS-CoV-2 and its pathophysiology was limited. Treatment protocols were primarily extrapolated from experiences with other coronaviruses such as SARS-CoV-1 (2003) and MERS-CoV (2012).
- Patients were managed with supportive care, and experimental use of antivirals like **lopinavir/ritonavir** and **hydroxychloroquine** was common, despite limited evidence.
- Oxygen therapy and mechanical ventilation were the mainstays for severe cases.

1.2 Challenges Faced

- **Diagnostic Delays:** Limited availability of RT-PCR testing led to delays in diagnosis.
- **Overburdened Healthcare Systems:** Hospitals were overwhelmed, and resources such as ventilators, oxygen, and personal protective equipment (PPE) were often insufficient.
- **High Mortality:** The absence of standardized protocols and effective treatments contributed to high case fatality rates in the early months.

AV.2 Mid-Pandemic: Evidence-Based Advances

2.1 Understanding the Disease Pathophysiology

- SARS-CoV-2 was identified to cause a biphasic illness:

1. **Viral Replication Phase**: Dominated by viral replication and symptoms like fever and cough.
2. **Hyperinflammatory Phase**: Characterized by a dysregulated immune response ("cytokine storm") leading to severe complications such as acute respiratory distress syndrome (ARDS) and multi-organ failure.

2.2 Key Therapeutic Breakthroughs

- **Corticosteroids:**
  - The **RECOVERY Trial** demonstrated the efficacy of **dexamethasone** in reducing mortality

in patients requiring oxygen or mechanical ventilation.

- This became a cornerstone of treatment for severe COVID-19. This was the first time that we started using corticosteroids to treat an infection

- **Antiviral Therapies:**
  - **Remdesivir** showed modest benefits in reducing the duration of hospitalization in patients with severe disease.
  - Favipiravir and molnupiravir were introduced for mild to moderate cases in certain countries, including India.
- **Immunomodulators:**
  - **Tocilizumab** (an IL-6 receptor antagonist) and **baricitinib** (a JAK inhibitor) were found to benefit patients with severe hyperinflammation.
- **Anticoagulation:**
  - The recognition of COVID-19-associated coagulopathy led to the widespread use of prophylactic and therapeutic anticoagulation to prevent thrombotic complications such as pulmonary embolism.
- **Oxygen Therapy Innovations:**
  - High-flow nasal cannula (HFNC) and non-invasive ventilation (NIV) were used to delay or avoid mechanical ventilation.

  - Prone positioning was shown to improve oxygenation in both ventilated and non-ventilated patients.

2.3 Vaccine Rollout

- As already described in detail, the development and deployment of vaccines marked a turning point in the pandemic.
- Vaccination significantly reduced the severity of disease, hospitalizations, and deaths.

AV.3 Late Pandemic: Personalized and Holistic Care

3.1 Evolving Therapies

- With the emergence of variants like Delta and Omicron, the efficacy of monoclonal antibodies (e.g., casirivimab/imdevimab) and antivirals was re-evaluated.
- Focus shifted to **booster vaccinations** to address waning immunity.

3.2 Long COVID Management

- **Post-Acute Sequelae of SARS-CoV-2 (PASC):**
  - Long COVID emerged as a major concern, with symptoms such as fatigue, dyspnea, and cognitive dysfunction persisting for months.
  - Multidisciplinary care was emphasized for rehabilitation.

3.3 Mental Health and Social Impact

- The pandemic highlighted the mental health burden on both patients and healthcare workers.
- Integrating psychological support into care became essential.

Reflections

Lessons Learned

a) **Rapid Knowledge Sharing**

- Collaborative efforts across nations and institutions enabled rapid data sharing and the establishment of evidence-based guidelines.
- Open-access platforms and preprint publications played a critical role.

b) **Preparedness is Crucial**

- Healthcare systems must be equipped with flexible infrastructures to handle surges in patient volumes.
- Stockpiling essential supplies (e.g., oxygen, PPE) is vital.

c) **Public Health Measures Work**

Non-pharmaceutical interventions (e.g., masking, social distancing) proved effective in reducing transmission.

d) **Vaccine Equity Matters**

Inequitable vaccine distribution highlighted the need for global cooperation to ensure fair access, especially in low-income countries.

e) **Adaptability in Medicine**

The pandemic underscored the importance of adaptability in clinical practice, with guidelines evolving based on emerging evidence.

The management of COVID-19 has evolved from experimental therapies and widespread uncertainty to evidence-based, personalized care. The pandemic has left an indelible mark on global health, teaching us the value of preparedness, collaboration, and resilience. As we move forward, the lessons learned must guide future responses to emerging infectious diseases to safeguard public health and ensure equitable care for all.

As this book goes to the press, China is currently experiencing a rise in cases of **human metapneumovirus (HMPV)**, a respiratory pathogen that typically causes symptoms akin to the common cold, such as cough, fever, nasal congestion, headache, and fatigue. While HMPV infections are generally mild, they can lead to more severe conditions like bronchiolitis or pneumonia, particularly in young children and immunocompromised individuals. Recent data from China's National Disease Control and Prevention Administration indicate an increase in HMPV infections among individuals under 14 years old, especially in northern provinces. Despite circulating unverified videos suggesting overwhelmed hospitals, Chinese authorities and the World Health Organization have not reported an outbreak of overwhelming magnitude. Foreign Ministry spokesperson Mao Ning noted that respiratory infections often peak during winter and assured that the government is attentive to public health, emphasizing that it remains safe to travel in China. In response to the uptick in respiratory illnesses, China has initiated a pilot program to monitor pneumonia cases of unknown origin, aiming to enhance preparedness for emerging pathogens during the winter season.

The buck should stop somewhere. A lot of mudslinging and evading responsibilities will continue. The saddest part is that whatever good habits humans adopted during the pandemic have already been forgotten. We have tried to document the para-pandemic events without being judgmental. We should not forget that "History repeats itself".

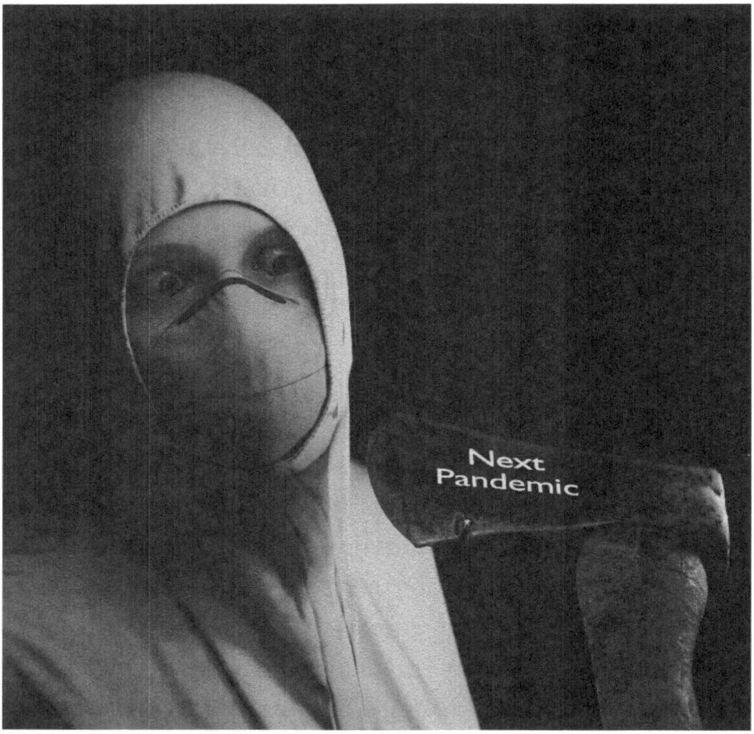

Are we ready for the next pandemic?

References

1. Dyer C. Patients launch legal action against AstraZeneca over its covid-19 vaccine,BMJ group. 2023;
2. Defoe D, Burgess A, Bristow C. A journal of the plague year. Modern Library; 1722.
3. Fenn EA. Pox americana: The great smallpox epidemic of 1775-82. Macmillan; 2002.
4. Foster JB, McChesney RW. The american empire: Pax americana or pox americana? Monthly Review. 2004;56(4):1–5.
5. Fletcher J. Camus, the liberation, and la peste: A fresh look. International Fiction Review. 1994;
6. Dhairyawan R. A shared COVID-19 testimony. The Lancet. 2021;397(10278):959–60.
7. Gilbert S, Green C, Crewe D. VAXXERS: The inside story of the oxford AstraZeneca vaccine and the race against the virus. CSIRO Publishing; 2021.
8. Rosen CS, Morland LA, Glassman LH, Marx BP, Weaver K, Smith CA, et al. Virtual mental health care in the veterans health administration's immediate response to coronavirus disease-19. American Psychologist. 2021;76(1):26.
9. Mandal S, Arinaminpathy N, Bhargava B, Panda S. Plausibility of a third wave of COVID-19 in india: A mathematical modelling based analysis. Indian Journal of medical research. 2021;153(5-6):522–32.
10. Morang'a CM, Ngoi JM, Gyamfi J, Amuzu DS, Nuertey BD, Soglo PM, et al. Genetic diversity of SARS-CoV-2 infections in ghana from 2020-2021. Nature Communications. 2022;13(1):2494.

11. Costa MJ. On saramago. JSTOR; 2013.
12. Karmakar G. Pandemic and man-less society: Problematizing gender, sex and sexuality in christina sweeney-baird's the end of men. In: Literary representations of pandemics, epidemics and pestilence. Routledge India; 2022. p. 43–51.
13. Hemingway E. MEN WITHOUT WOMEN: Ernest hemingway. Lebooks Editora; 2023.
14. Benchouk SK. From fiction to reality in steven soderbergh's contagion (2011), a prediction of coronavirus pandemic [PhD thesis]. university of Tlemcen; 2024.
15. Mandel ESJ. Station eleven. Éditions Rivages; 2016.
16. Kim D. Is asian or asian american viral?: Symptomatic relation between pandemic and global capitalism in ling ma's severance. 동서비교문학저널. 2023;(66):7–24.
17. Ali MI, Jannah SW, Pabur HE, Katili YAH. Thrilling encounters in social settings: A retelling of the eyes of darkness by dean koontz. Tamaddun. 2024;23(1):98–113.
18. Vijay K. Introductory chapter: The journey of vaccines-the past and the present. In: Vaccines-the history and future. IntechOpen; 2019.
19. Montagu LMW, Baron JASWM, et al. The letters and works of lady mary wortley montagu. Vol. 1. Carey, Lea & Blanchard; 1837.
20. Robbins Schug G, Blevins KE, Cox B, Gray K, Mushrif-Tripathy V. Infection, disease, and biosocial processes at the end of the indus civilization. PLoS One. 2013;8(12):e84814.
21. Riel-Salvatore J. Mad neanderthal disease? Some comments on" a potential role for transmissible spongiform encephalopathies in neanderthal extinction". Medical hypotheses. 2008;71(3):473–4.
22. Norrie P. A history of disease in ancient times: More lethal than war. Springer; 2016.

23. Cirillo VJ. Mariola espinosa, epidemic invasions: Yellow fever and the limits of cuban independence, 1878–1930, university of chicago press. Medical History. 2010;54(4):547–8.

24. Bristow N. American pandemic: The lost worlds of the 1918 influenza epidemic. Oxford University Press; 2012.

25. Packard RM. The making of a tropical disease: A short history of malaria. JHU Press; 2021.

26. Daschuk JW. Clearing the plains: Disease, politics of starvation and the loss of aboriginal life. University of Toronto Press; 2021.

27. Gleason EG. Faith, reason, and the plague in seventeenth-century tuscany. By carlo m. Cipolla. Ithaca, new york: Cornell university press, 1979. Church History. 1981;50(4):467–8.

28. McMillen CW. Pandemics: A very short introduction. Vol. 492. Oxford University Press; 2016.

29. Weiss HH. The SIR model and the foundations of public health. Materials matematics. 2013;0001–17.

30. He S, Peng Y, Sun K. SEIR modeling of the COVID-19 and its dynamics. Nonlinear dynamics. 2020;101:1667–80.

31. Cherian JP, Kizhakkethottam JJ. A technical assessment of SIR, SIR-v and SEIR epidemic models. In: 2023 IEEE international conference on recent advances in systems science and engineering (RASSE). IEEE; 2023. p. 1–7.

32. Peter O, Afolabi O, Victor A, Akpan C, Oguntolu F. Mathematical model for the control of measles. Journal of Applied Sciences and Environmental Management. 2018;22(4):571–6.

33. Mutalik AV. Models to predict H1N1 outbreaks: A literature review. Int J Community Med Public Health. 2017;4:3068–75.

34. Hay JA, Kennedy-Shaffer L, Kanjilal S, Lennon NJ, Gabriel SB, Lipsitch M, et al. Estimating epidemiologic dynamics from cross-sectional viral load distributions. Science. 2021;

35. Nadim SS, Chattopadhyay J. Occurrence of backward bifurcation and prediction of disease transmission with imperfect lockdown: A case study on COVID-19. Chaos, Solitons & Fractals. 2020;140:110163.

36. Castillo-Garsow CW, Castillo-Chavez C. A tour of the basic reproductive number and the next generation of researchers. In: An introduction to undergraduate research in computational and mathematical biology. Springer; 2020. p. 87–124.

37. Freeman WM, Walker SJ, Vrana KE. Quantitative RT-PCR: Pitfalls and potential. Biotechniques. 1999;26(1):112–25.

38. Pallen M. The last days of smallpox: Tragedy in birmingham. Epidemiology and Infection. 2018;147(e13):1–2.

39. Reardon S. NIH finds forgotten smallpox store. Nature. 2014;10.

40. Meselson M, Guillemin J, Hugh-Jones M, Langmuir A, Popova I, Shelokov A, et al. The sverdlovsk anthrax outbreak of 1979. Science. 1994;266(5188):1202–8.

41. Hu B, Guo H, Zhou P, Shi ZL. Characteristics of SARS-CoV-2 and COVID-19. Nature Reviews Microbiology. 2021;19(3):141–54.

42. Burrows W, Musteikis GM. Cholera infection and toxin in the rabbit ileal loop. The Journal of infectious diseases. 1966;183–90.

43. CHANG GG. NIH funded china's gain-of-function research at the wuhan institute of virology. 2021;

44. Potential "healthy vaccinee bias" in a study of BNT162b2 vaccine against covid-19. New England Journal of Medicine

[Internet]. 2023;389(3):284–6. Available from: https://doi.org/10.1056/NEJMc2306683

45. Kahn LH. One health and the politics of COVID-19. JHU Press; 2024.

46. Alasino E, Ramı□ rez MJ, Romero M, Schady N, Uribe D. Learning losses during the COVID-19 pandemic: Evidence from mexico. Economics of Education Review. 2024;98:102492.

47. Mogensen SW, Andersen A, Rodrigues A, Benn CS, Aaby P. The introduction of diphtheria-tetanus-pertussis and oral polio vaccine among young infants in an urban african community: A natural experiment. EBioMedicine. 2017;17:192–8.

48. Aaby P, Mogensen SW, Rodrigues A, Benn CS. Evidence of increase in mortality after the introduction of diphtheria–tetanus–pertussis vaccine to children aged 6–35 months in guinea-bissau: A time for reflection? Frontiers in public health. 2018;79.

49. Li C, Lee A, Grigoryan L, Arunachalam PS, Scott MK, Trisal M, et al. Mechanisms of innate and adaptive immunity to the pfizer-BioNTech BNT162b2 vaccine. Nature Immunology. 2022;23(4):543–55.

50. Visalli G, Laganà A, Lo Giudice D, Calimeri S, Caccamo D, Trainito A, et al. Towards a future of personalized vaccinology: Study on individual variables influencing the antibody response to the COVID-19 vaccine. Vaccines. 2023;11(2):217.

51. Sharma P, Kaur M, Narwal G. Other side of the COVID-19 pandemic: A review. Pharma Innov. 2020;9:366–9.

52. Olusola JA, Shote AA, Ouigmane A, Isaifan RJ. The impact of COVID-19 pandemic on nitrogen dioxide levels in Nigeria. PeerJ. 2021;9:e11387.

53. Kumar A, Singh P, Raizada P, Hussain CM. Impact of COVID-19 on greenhouse gases emissions: A critical review. Science of The Total Environment [Internet]. 2022;806:150349. Available from: https://www.sciencedirect.com/science/article/pii/S0048969721054267

54. Guevara M, Petetin H, Jorba O, Denier van der Gon H, Kuenen J, Super I, et al. European primary emissions of criteria pollutants and greenhouse gases in 2020 modulated by the COVID-19 pandemic disruptions. Earth System Science Data. 2022;14(6):2521–52.

55. Metya A, Dagupta P, Halder S, Chakraborty S, Tiwari YK, et al. COVID-19 lockdowns improve air quality in the south-east asian regions, as seen by the remote sensing satellites. Aerosol and Air Quality Research. 2020;20(8):1772–82.

56. Norrby E. Yellow fever and max theiler: The only nobel prize for a virus vaccine. The Journal of experimental medicine. 2007;204(12):2779–84.

57. Sridhar S. Clinical development of ebola vaccines. Therapeutic advances in vaccines. 2015;3(5-6):125–38.

58. Karikó K, Buckstein M, Ni H, Weissman D. Suppression of RNA recognition by toll-like receptors: The impact of nucleoside modification and the evolutionary origin of RNA. Immunity. 2005;23(2):165–75.

59. Matta A, Kunadharaju R, Osman M, Jesme C, McMiller Z, Johnson EM, et al. Clinical presentation and outcomes of myocarditis post mRNA vaccination: A meta-analysis and systematic review. Cureus. 2021;13(11).